SUZANNE JONES

BREAKING FREE From ARFID

A Compassionate Guide to Overcoming Eating Challenges

First edition

This book was professionally typeset on Reedsy.
Find out more at reedsy.com

Contents

Introduction

Welcome to "Breaking Free from ARFID: A Compassionate Guide to Overcoming Eating Challenges." If you or someone you care about struggles with Avoidant/Restrictive Food Intake Disorder (ARFID), you're in the right place. This book is here to offer understanding, practical help, and hope.

ARFID is more than just being a picky eater. It's a complex issue that affects your ability to eat a variety of foods, impacting both your body and mind. Living with ARFID can feel lonely and frustrating, but you are not alone. Many people face similar challenges, and there are ways to manage and overcome them.

In this book, we will explore ARFID in detail. You'll learn what it is, how it differs from other eating issues, and how it can affect people of all ages. We will talk about the physical and emotional effects of ARFID and provide practical tips for managing symptoms and improving your relationship with food.

This guide is designed to be clear and easy to follow. We'll break down complex ideas into simple terms, making sure you can easily understand and apply what you learn. We'll offer strategies for building a supportive network, setting achievable goals, and taking steps toward recovery.

Whether you have ARFID, support someone who does, or simply want to learn more, this book is here to help. Together, we will explore ways to overcome the challenges of ARFID and move toward a healthier, happier life.

Thank you for choosing this guide. Let's start this journey toward understanding, healing, and breaking free from ARFID.

I

Part 1: ARFID Unveiled

1

Chapter 1: Unveiling Avoidant Restrictive Food Intake Disorder (ARFID)

What is ARFID?

Avoidant Restrictive Food Intake Disorder (ARFID) is an eating disorder in which people avoid or restrict their food intake, resulting in serious health consequences. ARFID, unlike other eating disorders, is not motivated by concerns about body weight or appearance. Instead, it is caused by sensory sensitivities, a fear of negative outcomes such as choking or vomiting, or a general disinterest in eating.

Diagnostic Criteria

To diagnose ARFID, healthcare providers employ the following DSM-5 criteria.

- **Eating or eating disturbance:** This could include a lack of interest in eating, avoidance based on sensory aspects of food (such as texture, smell, or color), or fear of potential negative consequences of eating (such as choking). This disturbance causes a persistent failure to achieve adequate nutritional or energy needs, as shown by one or more of the following:

1. *Significant weight loss or failure to meet predicted weight increase in children.*
2. *Significant nutritional insufficiency.*
3. *Dependence on enteral (tube-fed) or oral dietary supplements.*
4. *Significant interference with daily activities, including social and psychological functioning.*

- **Not better explained by a lack of accessible food or culturally sanctioned practices:** The eating disorder should not be caused by a lack of available food or cultural practice that describes the restrictive eating behavior.
- **No body image disturbance:** The disorder is not limited to anorexia nervosa or bulimia nervosa, and it is not characterized by concerns about body weight or shape.
- **Not due to a concurrent physical ailment or another mental issue:** If the eating issue coexists with another illness or disorder, the severity of ARFID should surpass what is generally associated with that disease, necessitating additional professional attention.

History and Development of the ARFID Diagnosis

Avoidant Restrictive Food Intake Disorder (ARFID) is a relatively recent eating disorder that was officially recognized in the fifth edition of the Diagnostic and Statistical Manual of Mental Disorders (DSM-5) in 2013. The path to its acknowledgment reflects an increasing understanding of the diversity and complexity of eating behaviors.

Early observations

Historically, strange eating habits that did not meet the criteria for other eating disorders were frequently ignored or misdiagnosed. Children and adults who had strong dietary aversions or limits were sometimes labeled as "picky eaters" or diagnosed with infancy and early childhood feeding disorders. These diagnoses did not cover the entire complexity of the problem, especially when the behaviors continued beyond early childhood and resulted in significant nutritional deficits and psychosocial problems.

Recognizing the need for a new diagnosis

As doctors saw more patients with severely restricted eating that did not fit the traditional features of anorexia nervosa or bulimia nervosa, it became evident that a new diagnostic category was required. These individuals frequently lacked a preoccupation with body image or a fear of gaining weight, which are key characteristics of other eating disorders. Instead, their eating habits were motivated by sensory sensitivity, fear of negative repercussions, or a lack of interest in eating.

Development and Inclusion in DSM-5

The American Psychiatric Association (APA) saw the need for a diagnostic category that encompassed these distinct manifestations. Work on what would become ARFID began in earnest during the DSM-5 planning process. Researchers and physicians worked together to identify the illness and develop criteria that would distinguish it from other eating and feeding problems.

In 2013, ARFID was formally added to the DSM-5. This inclusion was an important step forward since it established a framework for diagnosis and therapy, allowing healthcare providers to better recognize and meet the needs of people with this disease.

Impact of the Diagnosis

The recognition of ARFID had a significant impact on the field of eating disorders. It has raised awareness among healthcare providers and the general public about the dangers of excessive dietary avoidance and restriction. With a precise diagnostic category, researchers can study ARFID more thoroughly, resulting in increased knowledge and treatment choices.

The creation of the ARFID diagnostic emphasizes the significance of recognizing and correcting various eating behaviors. It emphasizes that eating disorders are not one-size-fits-all and that a nuanced approach is required for accurate diagnosis and treatment. As awareness and understanding of ARFID spreads, more people will be able to receive the help and care they require to manage and overcome this difficult disorder.

Unveiling the Many Faces of ARFID

Avoidant Restrictive Food Intake Disorder (ARFID) can present in a variety of ways, reflecting the many reasons why people avoid or restrict their food intake. The three main manifestations are sensory aversions, fear of choking, and a lack of interest in food.

Sensory aversions

Many people with ARFID have significant sensory aversions to certain meals. These aversions are frequently linked to the texture, smell, taste, or appearance of specific meals. For example:

- **Texture:** Some people may avoid meals that are crunchy, slimy, or have a combination of textures because they find them unpleasant to consume.
- **Smell:** Strong odors can be unpleasant, thus people avoid foods with strong odors.
- **Taste:** Intense flavors, whether hot, bitter, or sweet, might cause aversion.
- **Appearance:** The color or shape of food can also be an important element, leading to avoiding unpleasant items.

These sensory sensitivities can significantly limit a person's willingness to eat a wide range of foods, frequently resulting in a highly restricted diet deficient in critical nutrients.

Fear of choking.

Another prevalent symptom of ARFID is fear of choking or vomiting. This fear may stem from a traumatic experience, such as a choking occurrence, or from concern about the possibility of choking or gagging while eating. Individuals experiencing this dread may:

- **Chew food excessively:** To ensure that it is completely broken down before swallowing.
- **Avoid certain textures:** Avoid foods with firm or crunchy textures, as these are perceived to be more likely to induce choking.
- **Limit your portion sizes:** To feel more in control of the eating process and less anxious.

The fear of choking can be crippling, resulting in significant weight loss and nutritional deficits as the spectrum of safe foods becomes progressively limited.

Lack of interest in food.

Some people with ARFID have a true disinterest in eating or food in general. This lack of interest is not due to body image issues but to a decreased appetite or indifference to eating. This presentation includes the following characteristics:

- **Minimal hunger cues:** Even after going for extended periods without eating, people may not feel hungry.
- **Limited pleasure from eating:** Food may not bring the same sensory gratification or enjoyment as it does to others.
- **Eating out of necessity:** Rather than for enjoyment, people may eat just because they have to, frequently in small quantities.

How ARFID Can Differ Across Age Groups

Avoidant Restrictive Food Intake Disorder (ARFID) affects people of all ages, however, the symptoms differ significantly between children and adults. Understanding the differences is essential for accurate diagnosis and treatment.

ARFID in Children

ARFID is frequently detected in children during their early childhood and might be misinterpreted for regular selective eating. However, ARFID is more severe and persistent than typical childhood picky eating behaviors.

Key Characteristics

- **Growth and Development Concerns:** Children with ARFID may have delayed growth and development due to inadequate nutrition. They may fail to acquire weight or grow at a normal rate for their age.
- **Dependence on Supplements:** Some children may require nutritional supplements or enteral feeding to meet their dietary needs.
- **Behavioral Signs:** Children may develop severe aversions to certain textures, tastes, or colors of food, resulting in tantrums or anxiety at mealtimes. They may also show indifference to food or eating.
- **Impact on Daily Life:** ARFID may interfere with social activities such as eating with peers or attending birthday parties, leading to feelings of loneliness or fear.

Treatment Approaches:

- **Behavioral Interventions:** Exposure treatment, for example, can help children gradually become more comfortable with other cuisines.
- **Parental Participation:** Educating and including parents in the therapeutic process is essential. Parents can learn techniques to encourage

and support their children's eating habits without putting them under pressure or creating negative food experiences.

- **Nutritional Support:** Working with a dietitian can help ensure that children receive the nutrients they require to develop and flourish.

ARFID for adults

Adult ARFID is often the outcome of unresolved childhood symptoms. However, it can arise later in life as a result of stress, trauma, or other factors.

Key Characteristics

- **Nutritional Deficiencies:** Adults with ARFID may suffer from nutritional deficits, leading to tiredness, impaired immune function, and anemia.
- **Psychosocial impact:** The condition can significantly impact social interactions and relationships. Adults may avoid food-related social gatherings, resulting in isolation and conflict in personal and professional relationships.
- **Mental Health Concerns:** In adults, ARFID is usually associated with anxiety, depression, and other mental health issues. The emotional cost might be high, affecting the overall quality of life.
- **Chronic Health Issues:** Long-term ARFID can lead to osteoporosis, cardiovascular problems, and gastrointestinal diseases.

Treatment Approaches:

- **Therapy Support:** Cognitive behavioral therapy (CBT) and other treatments can help individuals address the underlying psychological issues that contribute to ARFID. Exposure therapy can also help to gradually broaden the range of acceptable foods.
- **Nutritional Counselling:** A certified dietitian may assist adults with creating a balanced and diverse diet, correcting any nutritional deficiencies, and developing realistic stages to expand their food options.

- **Support Systems:** Encouraging adults to develop a support network, whether through family, friends, or support groups, can provide valuable motivation and understanding.

The Emotional Toll of ARFID

Avoidant Restrictive Food Intake Disorder (ARFID) can have significant emotional and psychological consequences. Aside from the physical health repercussions, people with ARFID frequently experience severe anxiety, melancholy, and humiliation, which can worsen their illness and impede rehabilitation.

Anxiety

Anxiety is commonly associated with ARFID. The condition itself can cause anxiety, and pre-existing anxiety problems can exacerbate ARFID symptoms.

Sources of Anxiety:

- **Food-related anxiety:** Many people with ARFID are extremely anxious about food. This might be caused by sensory sensitivities (for example, an aversion to textures or scents) or anxieties of choking or vomiting.
- **Social Anxiety:** Eating in public or social situations can be very uncomfortable. Fear of being judged or misunderstood by others might cause people to avoid social events involving eating, which contributes to social isolation.
- **Health-related anxiety:** Concerns regarding the physical health repercussions of ARFID, such as malnutrition or weight loss, can also be stressful.

Signs of Anxiety:

- **Physical Symptoms:** Increased heart rate, sweating, trembling, and gastrointestinal distress.
- **Behavioral Symptoms:** Avoidance of eating situations, reliance on safe foods, and ritualistic eating behaviors.

Depression

Depression is another major concern for many people with ARFID. The disorder's effects on daily living and social interactions might cause emotions of pessimism and sadness.

Contributing factors:

- **Isolation:** ARFID can cause loneliness and isolation, which are major risk factors for depression.
- **Frustration and Hopelessness:** Dealing with ARFID can be stressful and discouraging, especially when progress appears gradual or non-existent. This might lead to feelings of despondency and bad mood.
- **Negative Self-Perception:** Individuals with ARFID may acquire negative self-perceptions as a result of their eating behaviors, which can exacerbate depressive symptoms.

Symptoms of depression:

- **Emotional Symptoms:** Persistent sadness, hopelessness, and a lack of interest in previously enjoyed activities.
- **Physical Symptoms:** Changes in appetite or sleep patterns, fatigue, and difficulty concentrating.

Shame

Shame is a common and detrimental feeling connected with ARFID. Individuals with the illness frequently feel embarrassed or humiliated about their eating habits.

Sources of shame:

- **Stigma and Judgement:** Negative comments or judgments regarding people's eating habits can have a significant impact on those with ARFID. This may involve being labeled as "picky" or feeling misunderstood by those around them.
- **Internalized Stigma:** Over time, people may internalize cultural stigmas surrounding eating disorders, believing that their difficulties are a result of personal flaws rather than a real medical disease.

Effects of Shame:

- **Secrecy and Hiding:** Shame might cause individuals to hide their eating habits and avoid settings where they may be recognized or scrutinized.
- **Impact on Self-Esteem:** Persistent shame can significantly undermine self-esteem and self-worth, making it even more difficult to seek assistance and support.

The Impact of ARFID on Self-Esteem and Body Image

Avoidant Restrictive Food Intake Disorder (ARFID) can have a major impact on a person's self-esteem and body image, even if the disorder is not caused by weight or form concerns. ARFID's restrictive eating practices and social ramifications might result in negative self-esteem and body image issues.

Impact on self-esteem

Self-esteem describes how people perceive and regard themselves. Several reasons can contribute to low self-esteem in people with ARFID:

Social stigma and misunderstanding:

- **Negative Labels:** People with ARFID may be labeled as "picky eaters" or "difficult," which can be demeaning and harmful. Such designations might evoke feelings of inadequacy and shame.
- **Lack of comprehension:** A general lack of awareness and comprehension of ARFID can leave people feeling alone and misunderstood. They may struggle to explain their eating habits to others, resulting in irritation and low self-esteem.

Challenges in Daily Life:

- **Social Avoidance:** Avoiding social settings involving food might result in missed chances and feelings of exclusion. This avoidance might amplify feelings of loneliness and lower self-esteem.
- **Performance worry:** For both children and adults, the pressure to eat "normally" in front of others can cause tremendous stress and worry, undermining self-esteem.

Internal Struggle:

- **Self-criticism:** People with ARFID may blame themselves for their eating problems, considering their behavior as a personal failure rather than a medical issue. This self-criticism can be harsh and widespread, resulting in a chronically negative self-image.
- **Dissatisfaction with Progress:** Slow progress in extending dietary options or satisfying nutritional demands can cause dissatisfaction and feelings of defeat, lowering self-esteem.

Impact on Body Image

Body image in ARFID is a challenging topic. While the condition is not based on body image issues, the physical effects and societal pressures might influence how people perceive their bodies.

Physical consequences:

- **Nutritional deficiencies:** Inadequate nutrition can cause apparent physical changes such as weight loss, pale skin, hair loss, and other indicators of malnutrition. These changes can influence how people feel about their bodies.
- **Development Delays:** ARFID in children can cause development delays and failure to thrive, which may lead to body image issues as they compare themselves to their classmates.

Social Influences:

- **Cultural norms:** Individuals with ARFID may be influenced by societal norms around body size and eating habits. The pressure to conform to these norms can amplify negative sentiments about one's body and eating patterns.
- **Comparison to Peers:** Seeing peers engage in normal eating behaviors and achieve expected physical development can make people with ARFID feel strange or inadequate, affecting their body image.

Managing Self-Esteem and Body Image Issues

Therapeutic approaches:

- **Cognitive behavior therapy (CBT):** CBT can help people identify and challenge negative beliefs about themselves and their bodies, replacing them with more positive and realistic viewpoints.

- **Self-Compassion Training:** Techniques for developing self-compassion can be useful. Encouraging people to treat themselves with the same care they would give to a friend can boost self-esteem and body image.

Support systems:

- **Family and Friends:** Educating family and friends about ARFID can help create a supportive environment. Positive feedback and understanding from loved ones can improve self-esteem and create a healthy body image.
- **Support Groups:** Connecting with people who have had similar experiences can give you a sense of community and belonging, lowering feelings of loneliness and increasing self-esteem.

Positive self-care practices:

- **Mindfulness and meditation:** Mindfulness and meditation can help people become more tolerant and nonjudgmental of themselves and their bodies.
- **Celebrating Achievements:** Recognizing and celebrating modest accomplishments in ARFID management helps strengthen positive self-perception and boost confidence.

2

Chapter 2: ARFID vs. Picky Eating and Other Eating Disorders

Picky Eating or ARFID?

Picky eating is a widespread phenomenon, particularly among youngsters, marked by picky eating habits and a reluctance to try new foods. It is critical to identify picky eating from more serious eating disorders such as ARFID to guarantee adequate knowledge and treatment.

Features of Picky Eating

Picky eating usually entails the following behaviors:

Selective Eating:

- **Limited Food Choices:** Picky eaters frequently have a limited choice of items that they will eat. They may favor familiar foods and reject trying new or unexpected ones.
- **Preference for Certain Textures or Flavours:** Many fussy eaters have strong preferences for specific textures (e.g., crunchy, smooth) or flavours

(e.g., sweet, salty) and avoid foods that do not satisfy these standards.

Reluctance to Taste New Foods:

- **Neophobia:** Picky eaters frequently experience neophobia or the dread of sampling new foods. They may be cautious or even refuse to sample items they have never tried before.
- **Food Jags:** Picky eaters may go through periods in which they only desire to consume a specific food item and then abruptly reject it.

Mealtime Behaviours:

- **Prolonged Meal Times:** Picky eaters frequently take a long time to finish meals because they pick at them or eat slowly.
- **Avoidance Tactics:** Some picky eaters may use various strategies to avoid eating certain meals, such as making excuses or negotiating for alternative food options.

Differentiating between picky eating and ARFID.

While picky eating and ARFID have certain similarities, they differ in numerous important aspects.

Severity and Impact:

- **Nutritional Deficiency:** Picky eating, while annoying, typically does not result in serious nutritional shortages or significant weight loss. In contrast, ARFID can have major health effects, including as malnutrition and delayed growth.
- **Impact on Daily Life:** Picky eating rarely disrupts everyday tasks or social interactions. However, ARFID has a significant impact on social, educational, and occupational functioning.

Duration and Persistence:

- **Developmental Phase:** Picky eating is a common developmental period for many children, and it usually passes. ARFID, on the other hand, persists and does not resolve itself as the child grows older.

Underlying causes:

- **Behavioral patterns:** Picky eating is typically not associated with severe psychological distress or anxiety. ARFID, on the other hand, is frequently characterized by anxiety about eating, fear of choking, or high sensory sensitivity.

Response to Intervention:

- **Behavioral Modification:** Picky eaters frequently respond well to modest encouragement and exposure to a variety of meals. Interventions that make mealtime more enjoyable or involve children in food preparation can be helpful.
- **Therapeutic Needs:** People with ARFID often require more structured and extensive interventions, like as therapy, to address underlying anxiety and sensory difficulties.

Managing Picky Eating

Strategies for Parents and Carers:

- **Patience and persistence:** Encourage your children to try different meals without forcing them. A youngster may need several exposures to a new cuisine before accepting it.
- **Positive Role Modelling:** Showcase healthy eating habits and an openness to trying new foods.

- **Participation in Food Preparation:** Involve finicky eaters in meal planning and preparation to improve their interest in new foods.
- **Creating a Positive Mealtime Environment:** Refrain from pressuring or scolding youngsters for not eating. Instead, make eating a relaxing and delightful experience.

Nutritional guidance:

- **Balanced food:** Make sure the child's food is balanced, even if it is limited, to avoid nutritional deficits. A pediatrician or dietitian can offer advice on meeting nutritional requirements.
- **Gradual Introduction of New Foods:** New foods should be introduced gradually and paired with established favorites to make them more enticing.

Comparing and Contrasting the Characteristics of ARFID and Picky Eating

Understanding the distinctions and similarities between Avoidant Restrictive Food Intake Disorder (ARFID) and picky eating is critical for proper diagnosis and treatment. While both include selective eating behaviors, they differ greatly in severity, underlying reasons, and effects on daily living.

Similarities

Selective Eating Patterns:

- **Limited Food Range:** ARFID and fussy eating both have a limited range of acceptable foods. Individuals may choose familiar foods while avoiding new or diversified options.
- **Strong Food Preferences:** In either situation, there may be a predilection for specific textures, flavours, or types of food.

Avoiding New Foods:

- **Food Neophobia:** Both ARFID and picky eaters frequently experience neophobia, which is the fear of trying new foods, resulting in hesitation or unwillingness to eat unfamiliar foods.

Differences

Severity and impact:

- **Nutritional Impact:** Picky eating rarely causes significant nutritional shortages or serious health repercussions. In contrast, ARFID can cause substantial health problems including malnutrition, developmental delays in children, and significant weight loss in adults.
- **Daily Functioning:** While picky eating can cause occasional mealtime issues, it rarely interferes with daily activities. However, the anxiety and limits imposed by ARFID can have a significant influence on social interactions, educational involvement, and vocational functioning.

Psychological and emotional factors:

- **Emotional Distress:** Individuals with ARFID frequently suffer worry, dread, and emotional distress while eating, such as fear of choking or vomiting. Picky eaters are less likely to experience mental distress as a result of their eating habits.
- **Mental Health Associations:** ARFID is frequently associated with other mental health difficulties, including anxiety disorders, depression, and obsessive-compulsive disorder. While picky eating might be annoying, it is not often related to these psychological problems.

Duration and Development:

- **Persistence Over Time:** Picky eating is a common developmental stage that many youngsters go through before outgrowing. ARFID is a chronic disorder that does not improve with age and can last until adulthood if not treated.

- **Age of Onset:** Picky eating typically begins in early childhood and may improve with time. ARFID can also occur in childhood, but it usually persists unless treated properly.

Behavioural responses:

- **Behavioral Signs:** Picky eaters may be resistant to eating new foods, but they will eat enough to stay healthy and grow. Individuals with ARFID may demonstrate severe avoidance behaviours, such as gagging, vomiting, or intense distress at the sight or scent of specific foods.
- **Response to Intervention:** Behavioural tactics such as positive reinforcement, making mealtime interesting, and including children in food preparation are frequently effective for picky eating. ARFID is often treated with more intense and systematic therapies, such as cognitive-behavioral therapy (CBT) and exposure therapy.

Professional Evaluation and Treatment:

- **Need for Professional Assistance:** Picky eating can frequently be controlled with parental strategies and simple dietary supervision. ARFID, given its severity and severe health consequences, necessitates a professional examination and a thorough treatment plan that includes therapists, nutritionists, and, in certain cases, medical experts.

The Importance of a Professional Evaluation

When dealing with eating behaviors that may indicate Avoidant Restrictive Food Intake Disorder (ARFID) or other serious eating disorders, it is critical to get professional help. A full evaluation can distinguish between normal picky eating and more significant diseases such as ARFID, ensuring accurate diagnosis and treatment.

Accurate diagnosis.

Understanding symptoms:

- **Detailed Assessment:** Professionals undertake detailed assessments to determine the complete range of symptoms. This encompasses eating habits, psychological considerations, and physical health outcomes.
- **Differential Diagnosis:** A professional can separate ARFID from other eating disorders, such as anorexia nervosa, as well as from regular fussy eating. This ensures that the appropriate condition is diagnosed and treated.

Comprehensive Evaluation:

- **Medical History:** A detailed medical history will assist detect any underlying health issues that may be causing dietary difficulties.
- **Psychological Assessment:** Evaluating psychological health is critical for identifying any co-occurring mental health conditions, such as anxiety or depression, which may exacerbate eating disorders.
- **Nutritional Analysis:** Measuring dietary consumption and nutritional status can assist assess the severity of any deficits or malnutrition.

Tailored Treatment Plan

Individualized Approach:

- **Personalized Interventions: A** professional evaluation helps create a treatment plan tailored to the individual's needs. This could involve cognitive-behavioral therapy (CBT), exposure treatment, and nutritional counselling.

- **Multidisciplinary Team:** To provide holistic care, a comprehensive treatment plan frequently includes a team of professionals such as therapists, dietitians, and medical doctors.

Behavioural strategies:

- **Therapeutic strategies:** Professionals can use evidence-based therapeutic strategies to assist people in gradually broadening their food repertoire and lessen anxiety about eating.
- **Nutritional Advice:** A licensed dietitian can design a balanced meal plan that fits the individual's nutritional requirements while taking into account their dietary preferences and aversions.

Monitoring & Support

Ongoing Assessment:

- **Regular Monitoring:** Professional evaluation guarantees continuous monitoring of progress and allows for revisions to the treatment plan as needed. This is critical for dealing with any setbacks or obstacles that arise during the rehabilitation process.
- **Assistance and Guidance:** Continuous assistance from healthcare experts reassures and motivates individuals and families, allowing them to stick to the treatment plan.

Early Intervention:

- **Preventing Complications:** Early detection and intervention can help prevent severe nutritional shortages, growth delays, and other health problems linked with ARFID.
- **Better Outcomes:** The sooner ARFID is correctly recognized and treated,

the better the results. Early intervention has the potential to greatly enhance the quality of life and general health of those with ARFID.

Family and Carers' Education

Informed Support:

- **Educating Families:** Professional evaluation includes educating family and carers about ARFID to assist them in understanding the disorder and properly supporting their loved ones.
- **Building a Supportive atmosphere:** Knowledgeable families may establish a pleasant and encouraging atmosphere that promotes recovery and lessens the stigma associated with eating disorders.

Community Resources:

- **Access to Resources:** Professionals can connect individuals and their families with support groups, community resources, and advocacy organizations that give further help and information.

Understanding the Similarities and Differences Between ARFID and Other Eating Disorders

Avoidant restricted Food Intake Disorder (ARFID) and Anorexia Nervosa are both eating disorders that entail restricted eating behaviors, but they have quite different underlying causes, motivations, and effects on individuals. Understanding these similarities and distinctions is critical to accurate diagnosis and therapy.

Similarities

Restricted Eating Patterns:

- **Limited dietary Intake:** Both ARFID and Anorexia Nervosa need severe dietary restriction, which can result in malnutrition, weight loss, and a variety of health issues.
- **Nutritional Deficiencies:** Individuals with both illnesses are at risk of nutritional deficits due to their restricted diets. This can cause similar physical symptoms, such as weariness, dizziness, and reduced immunity.

Health consequences:

- **Physical Health Risks:** Both disorders can cause serious physical health issues, such as compromised immune systems, developmental delays in children, and significant organ damage.
- **Psychological Distress:** Individuals with ARFID and Anorexia Nervosa frequently feel severe psychological distress as a result of their eating behaviors. Anxiety and depression are prevalent in both disorders.

Need for Professional Intervention:

- **Comprehensive Treatment:** To address the complex interplay of physical and mental health difficulties, both disorders require expert intervention, such as medical monitoring, nutritional counseling, and psychological therapy.

Differences

Underlying causes and motivations:

Motivation for Restriction:

- **ARFID:** The primary motivation for food avoidance in ARFID is not body image or the fear of weight gain. Instead, it is generally caused by sensory sensitivities, fear of unpleasant outcomes (such as choking or vomiting), or a lack of enthusiasm for eating.
- **Anorexia Nervosa:** Anorexia Nervosa, on the other hand, is driven mostly by a fear of gaining weight and a distorted body image. Individuals restrict their food consumption to control their weight and shape, frequently motivated by a desire to achieve an unrealistic body ideal.

Emotional Triggers:

- **ARFID:** Emotional triggers in ARFID are generally associated with fears or sensory experiences related to eating. For example, a previous choking experience can cause a phobia of swallowing.
- **Anorexia Nervosa:** Emotional triggers in Anorexia Nervosa are typically associated with body dissatisfaction and a desire for thinness. Social pressures, cultural notions of beauty, and personal self-esteem concerns all play important roles.

Age of onset and demographics:

Age of Onset:

- **ARFID:** ARFID usually appears in early childhood and can persist into adulthood if not treated. It is not unusual for symptoms to appear during toddlerhood or early childhood.
- **Anorexia Nervosa:** Anorexia Nervosa typically begins in youth or young adulthood, however it can occur at any age. The peak onset normally occurs between the ages of 15 and 19.

Demographics:

- **ARFID:** ARFID affects both men and women, with no clear gender bias.

It is recognized across all age groups and is not always associated with cultural pressures on body appearance.

- **Anorexia Nervosa:** Anorexia Nervosa primarily affects women, though men can also be afflicted. The illness is more widespread in Western societies, which place a high value on thinness and body image.

Behavioural signs:

Behavioral Patterns:

- **ARFID:** Individuals with ARFID may avoid particular meals due to texture, color, or smell, and have strict eating habits. They may also avoid food due to specific anxieties, such as choking.
- **Anorexia Nervosa:** Individuals suffering from anorexia nervosa frequently engage in weight-controlling behaviors such as excessive exercise, calorie counting, and avoiding high-calorie foods. They may also engage in behaviors like body checking or wearing loose clothing to disguise their weight reduction.

Psychological characteristics:

Body Image:

- **ARFID:** Individuals with ARFID often do not have concerns about their body image. Their eating habits are not driven by a desire to be skinny or to maintain their weight.
- **Anorexia Nervosa:** Anorexia Nervosa is characterized by distorted body image. Individuals frequently see themselves as overweight, even if they are underweight, and are concerned about their physical shape and size.

ARFID vs. Avoidant/Restrictive Food Intake Disorder (ARFID) in the Context of Anorexia Nervosa

Avoidant/Restrictive Food Intake Disorder (ARFID) and Anorexia Nervosa are both severe eating disorders, although they differ greatly in their clinical presentation, underlying motivations, and psychological characteristics. However, there may be aspects of avoidant or restrictive eating in Anorexia Nervosa that resemble ARFID. Understanding the intricacies is critical for accurate diagnosis and therapy.

ARFID

Definition and Characteristics:

- **Non-Weight Related Motivations:** ARFID is defined by restricted eating habits that are not motivated by worries about weight or body form. Instead, these behaviors are caused by sensory sensitivities, a fear of undesirable outcomes (such as choking or vomiting), or a lack of desire to eat.
- **Sensory Aversions:** People with ARFID may avoid specific meals because of their texture, flavor, smell, or appearance.
- **Fear-Based Avoidance:** People may avoid eating because they are afraid of choking, vomiting, or having other unpleasant experiences.
- **Lack of Interest:** Some people with ARFID have no interest in food or eating, which can lead to inadequate intake.
- **Nutritional deficits:** ARFID's restrictive eating practices frequently result in nutritional deficits, weight loss, or inability to meet predicted weight increases in children.

Psychological Impact:

- **Anxiety and Distress:** Anxiety and distress are frequently associated with eating or anticipating eating, although they are unrelated to body image or weight worries.

- **Social and Emotional Consequences:** The illness can have a substantial influence on social relationships and daily functioning, as mealtimes become unpleasant.

Anorexia Nervosa

Definition and Characteristics.

- **Weight-Related Motivations:** Anorexia Nervosa is characterized by a strong fear of gaining weight and a distorted body image. Individuals with this disease aggressively restrict their food intake to maintain their weight.
- **Restrictive Eating:** This can include rigorous calorie counting, avoiding high-calorie items, and following stringent eating plans.
- **Excessive Exercise:** People may engage in excessive physical exercise to burn calories and reduce weight.
- **Body Image Distortion:** A key feature of Anorexia Nervosa is a considerable distortion in how people view their body size and shape, with many seeing themselves as overweight despite being underweight.

Psychological Impact:

- **Fear of Weight Gain:** The fear of gaining weight or becoming fat motivates restrictive eating habits and other weight-control methods.
- **Perfectionism and Control:** There is frequently an element of perfectionism and a need for control that transcends beyond eating behaviors and into other aspects of life.
- **Co-occurring Disorders:** Anorexia Nervosa is frequently accompanied by anxiety, depression, and obsessive-compulsive behavior.

ARFID-like Behaviours of Anorexia Nervosa

Overlap in behaviors:

- **Avoidance and Restriction:** ARFID and Anorexia Nervosa share avoidant and restrictive eating behaviors. However, the motivations for these behaviors vary greatly.
- **Fear-Based Avoidance:** While ARFID involves avoidance due to anxieties of undesirable physical consequences (such as choking), those suffering from Anorexia Nervosa may develop avoidant behaviors out of fear of gaining weight.

Differentiating Factors:

- **Primary Motivation:** The primary motivation is the most important differentiator. In ARFID, avoidance is motivated by sensory difficulties, fear of negative repercussions, or a lack of interest in food. Anorexia Nervosa's major motive is a strong fear of gaining weight and a desire to be slim.
- **Body Image Issues:** Body image distortion and the fear of gaining weight are important to Anorexia Nervosa, but not in ARFID.
- **Therapeutic Approach:** Treatment for ARFID focuses on addressing specific fears or sensory sensitivities and improving nutritional intake, whereas treatment for Anorexia Nervosa addresses distorted body image, and fear of weight gain, and frequently includes interventions for co-occurring psychological issues.

Co-occurrence:

- **Complex cases:** In very severe circumstances, an individual with Anorexia Nervosa may display ARFID-like behaviors, such as acute sensitivity to food textures or a fear of choking. However, these behaviors are usually considered secondary to the major problem of weight gain.

- **Holistic Treatment:** Individuals with features of both illnesses require a comprehensive treatment strategy that addresses all elements of their eating habits and psychological well-being.

ARFID vs. Other Restrictive Eating Disorders

Avoidant/Restrictive Food Intake Disorder (ARFID) and other restrictive eating disorders have some characteristics, particularly in terms of food avoidance and restriction. However, they differ greatly in terms of underlying motivations, psychological traits, and health consequences. Understanding these distinctions is critical for proper diagnosis and therapy.

Similarities

Restricted Eating Patterns:

- **Limited Food Intake:** Both ARFID and other restrictive eating disorders need considerable food restrictions, which can lead to malnutrition and other health issues.
- **Nutritional Deficiencies:** Individuals with ARFID and other restrictive eating disorders are at risk of nutritional deficiencies, which can cause exhaustion, decreased immunity, and growth problems.

Health consequences:

- **Physical Health Risks:** Both diseases can lead to serious physical health consequences, such as stunted growth and development, especially in children and teenagers.
- **Psychological Distress:** Anxiety and psychological distress associated with eating behaviors are prevalent in both ARFID and other restrictive eating disorders.

Need for Professional Intervention:

- **Comprehensive therapy:** ARFID and other restrictive eating disorders necessitate a comprehensive approach to therapy that includes medical, nutritional, and psychological interventions.

Differences

Underlying motivations:

ARFID:

- **Sensory Sensitivities:** People with ARFID may avoid certain foods because of sensory difficulties such as texture, taste, smell, or appearance.
- **Fear of Negative Consequences:** There may be a strong fear of adverse physical reactions such as choking, vomiting, or allergies.
- **Lack of Interest:** Some people with ARFID exhibit a general disinterest in food or eating that is unrelated to worries about body weight or shape.

Other restrictive eating disorders:

- **Body Image Concerns:** Disorders such as Anorexia Nervosa and Bulimia Nervosa are characterized by a strong fear of gaining weight and a distorted body image. Individuals limit their food consumption to maintain their weight and shape.
- **Emotional and psychological factors:** Low self-esteem, perfectionism, and a craving for control are common underpinnings of these diseases. Restrictive eating may be used as a coping method to alleviate emotional pain.
- **Cultural and social influences:** Societal pressures and cultural ideals of thinness and beauty have a substantial impact on the development and persistence of diseases such as Anorexia Nervosa.

Age of onset and demographics:

ARFID:

- **Early Onset:** ARFID typically begins in childhood and can last throughout adulthood if not handled. It affects both men and women quite equally.
- **Non-Weight Related:** ARFID is unaffected by cultural demands around body appearance or weight.

Other restrictive eating disorders:

- **Adolescence and Young Adulthood:** Disorders such as Anorexia Nervosa and Bulimia Nervosa usually appear throughout adolescence or young adulthood. They are more common in women, but can also afflict men.
- **Weight and Body Image Issues:** These disorders are largely impacted by cultural and societal expectations of thinness and attractiveness.

Behavioural signs:

ARFID:

- **Selective Eating:** ARFID can lead to selective eating when individuals avoid certain meals due to sensory qualities and have a limited range of "safe" items to consume.
- **Mealtime Stress:** Eating certain foods might cause severe worry or distress.

Other restrictive eating disorders:

- **Extreme Dieting:** Some people engage in extreme dieting behaviors, such as excessive calorie restriction, food avoidance, and inflexible eating habits.
- **Compensatory Behaviors:** Individuals with illnesses like Bulimia Ner-

vosa may engage in compensatory behaviors such as purging, excessive exercise, or the use of laxatives to regulate their weight.

Psychological characteristics:

ARFID:

- **Non-Weight Related Anxiety:** In ARFID, anxiety and distress are not related to body weight or shape, but rather to the act of eating specific foods.
- **Behavioral Rigidity:** There may be a strict adherence to specific eating habits or food preferences.

Other restrictive eating disorders:

- **Distorted Body Image:** Anorexia Nervosa is characterized by a distorted body image and an excessive dread of gaining weight.
- **Emotional Regulation:** Restrictive eating behaviors are often used to regulate emotions and establish control over one's life.

When to Seek Professional Help: Recognizing the Signs of ARFID

Recognizing the early signs and symptoms of Avoidant/Restrictive Food Intake Disorder (ARFID) is critical for effective diagnosis and treatment. While the presentation of ARFID varies by individual, certain red flags and warning indicators are similar in both children and adults. Understanding these symptoms can assist carers, educators, and healthcare professionals in recognizing the problem and seeking appropriate treatment.

Common Red Flags in Children

Selective Eating:

- **Food Restrictions:** A child's willingness to eat only a limited number of foods, often avoiding entire food groups.
- **Strong Preferences:** Extreme preferences for certain textures, colors, or food kinds (for example, only eating crunchy or bland foods).

Sensory sensitivities:

- **Aversion to Textures:** A refusal to consume meals with specific textures, such as soft, mushy, or mixed textures.
- **Smell Sensitivity:** Strong sensitivities to the smell of specific meals, resulting in avoidance.

Fear-Based Avoidance:

- **Fear of Choking or Vomiting:** Expressing concern or anxiety about choking, vomiting, or other unpleasant eating events.
- **Previous Trauma:** Avoiding certain foods following a traumatic experience, such as choking or an allergic response.

Lack of Interest in Eating:

- **Reduced Appetite:** Consistent lack of appetite or interest in eating.
- **Prolonged Mealtimes:** Eating for an exceptionally lengthy time or expressing anxiety during meals.

Physical Symptoms:

- **weight loss or poor growth:** Failure to acquire weight or grow as predicted can result in developmental problems.

- **Nutritional Deficiencies:** signs of malnutrition such as weariness, pallor, and recurrent illness.

Behavioral Signs:

- **Routine and Rituals:** Rigid mealtime routines and rituals, such as requiring precise food preparation or eating times.
- **Avoidance of Social Eating:** The unwillingness or inability to engage in meals at school, family events, or restaurants.

Common Red Flags in Adults

Restrictive Eating Patterns:

- **Narrow Food Choices:** Consistently consuming a small variety of foods while avoiding new or unfamiliar ones.
- **Rigid Eating Habits:** Sticking to tight eating patterns and routines with limited flexibility.

Sensory and fear-related issues:

- **Texture and Smell Sensitivity:** Avoiding foods because of texture or smell aversions, which may be related to sensory processing difficulties.
- **Fear of Adverse Reactions:** An ongoing fear of choking, vomiting, or experiencing an allergic reaction while eating.

Lack of interest in food:

- **Decreased Appetite:** A persistent lack of interest in food or eating, typically resulting in insufficient calorie intake.
- **Monotonous Diet:** Relying on a limited number of "safe" foods while

avoiding dietary variety.

Physical Health Concerns:

- **Weight Loss:** Inadvertent weight loss or difficulties maintaining a healthy weight.
- **Health Complications:** starvation symptoms such as dizziness, hair loss, and decreased immunity.

Psychosocial Impact:

- **Social Withdrawal:** Avoidance of social events involving eating, such as dining out with friends or attending social parties.
- **Emotional anguish:** Severe anxiety or anguish associated with eating, which can influence general mental health and well-being.

Behavioural signs:

- **Mealtime Rituals:** Performing precise rituals or routines during meals, such as chopping food into little pieces or eating in a set order.
- **Compensatory Behaviors:** Excessive use of supplements or meal replacements to avoid eating conventional foods.

The Importance of Early Intervention

Early intervention in Avoidant/Restrictive Food Intake Disorder (ARFID) is critical to avoiding long-term physical, emotional, and psychological repercussions. Recognizing the symptoms and receiving expert care as soon as possible can considerably enhance the quality of life for people who suffer from this illness. Here's why early intervention is so important.

Physical Health Benefits

Prevention of malnutrition:

- **Nutrient Intake:** Early intervention ensures that individuals acquire the nutrients their bodies require. Proper nutrition is essential for development, vitality, and good health.
- **Growth and Development:** Addressing ARFID early can help children and adolescents avoid growth delays and developmental difficulties, allowing them to attain their full potential.

Avoiding Severe Health Complications:

- **Long-term Health Risks:** Prolonged dietary shortages can cause serious health problems such as reduced immune systems, anemia, and bone density loss. Early action can help to mitigate these hazards.
- **Chronic issues:** Treating ARFID early lowers the chance of developing chronic health issues associated with inadequate nutrition, such as cardiovascular disease and osteoporosis.

Emotional and Psychological Benefits

Reducing Anxiety and Depression:

- **Mental Health:** Early treatment might help control the anxiety and depression that are commonly associated with ARFID. Effective therapy interventions can increase emotional well-being while also reducing eating-related distress.
- **Improved Self-Esteem:** Addressing ARFID early on can help people develop a healthier connection with food and their bodies, increasing self-esteem and confidence.

Developing Healthy Eating Habits:

- **Behavioral Changes:** Early intervention enables people to adopt healthy eating habits before restrictive patterns become thoroughly ingrained. This makes it easy to broaden food choices and boost overall nutrition.
- **Positive Mealtime Experiences:** Early intervention can make mealtimes less stressful and pleasurable, establishing a positive attitude towards food and eating.

Social and Relational Benefits

Enhanced Social Interaction:

- **Social Participation:** Early therapy makes people more comfortable in social interactions including eating, reducing isolation, and improving social ties.
- **Supportive Relationships:** Involving family and friends in early intervention helps to promote understanding and encouragement throughout the healing process.

Improved Family Dynamics:

- **Family Involvement:** Early intervention with family-based therapy can improve family dynamics by educating members about ARFID and providing support techniques. This can enhance family interactions and lessen conflict over food concerns.

Academic and Occupational Benefits

Improved Academic Performance:

- **Concentration and Energy:** A good diet is critical for cognitive function, concentration, and energy levels. Addressing ARFID early can improve academic achievement by ensuring that people get enough nutrition to support their learning and growth.
- **Attendance and engagement:** Less worry and greater physical health contribute to increased school attendance and engagement in activities, resulting in a more rewarding educational experience.

Enhanced Occupational Functioning:

- **Work Performance:** Early intervention can improve people's occupational functioning by treating physical and emotional issues that hinder job performance.
- **Professional Relationships:** Lowering anxiety about eating can improve professional relationships and participation in work-related social events.

Long-term outcomes

Sustained Recovery:

- **Early Success:** Early intervention increases the likelihood of successful treatment outcomes, reduces the risk of relapse, and promotes long-term recovery.
- **Resilience Building:** Learning coping methods and having a healthy relationship with food early on increases resilience, allowing people to manage future problems more effectively.

Quality of life:

- **Overall Well-Being:** Treating ARFID early improves people's overall well-being, helping them to live healthier, happier, and more satisfying lives.
- **Complication Prevention:** Early therapy prevents symptoms and com-

plications from worsening, lowering ARFID's long-term impact on a person's life.

II

Part 2: How ARFID Impacts Your Life

3

Chapter 3: The Physical Health Consequences of ARFID

Malnutrition and its Devastating Impact on the Body

Avoidant/Restrictive Food Intake Disorder (ARFID) can cause serious nutrient deficits due to a limited variety of foods consumed. These inadequacies can have a significant impact on physical health, development, and well-being. Here, we will look at the most frequent nutrient deficiencies linked with ARFID, their symptoms, and the necessity of addressing them early on with nutritional support.

Common Nutrient Deficits

1. Protein:

- **Role in the Body:** Proteins' role in the body includes growth, muscle development, immunological function, and cell repair and maintenance.
- **Symptoms of Deficiency:** muscle atrophy, weariness, a compromised immune system, and slower wound healing.
- **Sources:** meat, poultry, fish, eggs, dairy products, legumes, nuts, and

45

seeds.

2. Iron:

- **Role in the Body:** Iron is essential for producing hemoglobin, which transports oxygen in the blood, and for energy metabolism.
- **Symptoms of Deficiency:** Anemia, weariness, weakness, pale skin, shortness of breath, and dizziness.
- **Sources:** Red meat, chicken, fish, lentils, beans, spinach, and iron-fortified cereals.

3. Calcium:

- **Role in the Body:** Calcium is vital for bone health, muscle function, nerve transmission, and blood clotting.
- **Symptoms of Deficiency:** Osteoporosis, brittle bones, muscle spasms, and tingling in the fingers.
- **Sources:** Dairy products, fortified plant-based milk, leafy green vegetables, tofu, and almonds.

4. Vitamin D:

- **Role in the Body:** Promotes calcium absorption, bone health, and immunological function, and reduces inflammation.
- **Symptoms of Deficiency:** Bone discomfort, muscle weakness, an increased risk of fractures, and weariness.
- **Sources:** Sun exposure, fatty fish, fortified dairy products, and supplements.

5.Vitamin B12:

- **Role in the Body:** Vitamin B12 is essential for red blood cell development, brain function, and DNA synthesis.

- **Symptoms of Deficiency:** Anemia, weariness, weakness, nerve damage, memory loss, and cognitive impairment.
- **Sources:** Meat, fish, poultry, eggs, dairy products, and fortified cereals.

6. Zinc:

- **Role in the Body:** Zinc promotes immunological function, wound healing, DNA synthesis, and cell division.
- **Symptoms of Deficiency:** Impaired immunological response, poor wound healing, hair loss, and lack of appetite.
- **Sources:** Meat, seafood, beans, seeds, nuts, and dairy products.

7. Essential Fatty Acids:

- **Role in the Body:** Essential fatty acids, such as omega-3 and omega-6 are crucial for brain function, reducing inflammation, and maintaining heart health.
- **Symptoms of Deficiency:** Dry skin, hair loss, poor wound healing, and cognitive issues.
- **Sources:** Fatty fish, flaxseed, chia seeds, walnuts, and plant oils.

Importance of Addressing Nutrient Deficits

1. Physical Health :

- **Growth and Development:** Adequate nutrition is essential for growth and development, especially in children and adolescents. Nutrient deficits can cause stunted growth and developmental disabilities.
- **Immune Function:** Proper nutrition boosts the immune system, lowering the likelihood of infection and sickness. Nutrient deficits can impair the immune system, making people more vulnerable to disease.

2. Cognitive and Emotional Wellbeing:

- **Cognitive Function:** Iron, vitamin B12, and essential fatty acids are critical nutrients for brain health and cognition. Deficits can affect learning, memory, and concentration.
- **Emotional Well-Being:** Nutrient deficiencies can lead to mood disorders including anxiety and despair. Adequate eating promotes mental health and emotional stability.

3. Long-Term Health:

- **Chronic Disease Prevention:** Addressing vitamin deficiencies can avoid chronic diseases like osteoporosis, cardiovascular disease, and anemia.
- **Quality of Life:** Providing enough nourishment increases overall quality of life, allowing people to participate more fully in daily activities and social interactions.

Strategies to Address Nutrient Deficiencies

1. Professional Evaluation:

- **Comprehensive Assessment:** A comprehensive assessment by healthcare professionals, such as a registered dietitian and physicians, is crucial for identifying particular nutrient deficits and developing a personalized treatment plan.
- **Nutritional evaluating:** Regularly evaluating nutritional status allows you to track your progress and make adjustments to your treatment plan as needed.

2. Dietary Interventions:

- **Balanced Meal Plans:** Creating balanced meal plans with nutrient-dense foods helps correct deficits and guarantee optimal nutrition intake.

- **Safe Food Exploration:** Gradually introducing new foods and broadening the definition of "safe" foods helps increase dietary variety and nutrient intake.

3. Supplementation:

- **Targeted Supplements:** When dietary adjustments are insufficient, supplementing with specific nutrients (e.g., iron, vitamin D, vitamin B12) can help resolve deficiencies.
- **Practitioner Advice:** Supplements should be taken under the supervision of a healthcare practitioner to avoid over-supplementation and potential negative effects.

The Impact of Malnutrition on Growth and Development

Malnutrition is a major complication of Avoidant/Restrictive Food Intake Disorder (ARFID), affecting both physical growth and developmental milestones. Understanding these effects is critical for recognizing the value of early intervention and complete therapy for people with ARFID.

Physical Growth

1. Stunted Growth:

- **Height and Weight:** Malnutrition can cause stunted growth, resulting in shorter and lighter youngsters compared to their contemporaries. Adequate nutrition is especially important during periods of fast growth, such as infancy, youth, and adolescence.
- **Delayed Puberty:** Inadequate nutritional intake can cause puberty to occur later, impacting the physical development involved with this essential stage of life.

2. Bone Health:

- **Bone Density:** Optimal bone density requires calcium and vitamin D. Malnutrition can weaken bones, increasing the risk of fractures and osteoporosis later in life.
- **Growth Plates:** Proper nutrition helps the growth plates in bones, which are required for bone lengthening and overall growth. Malnutrition can cause these plates to close prematurely, preventing growth.

3. Muscle Development:

- **Muscle Mass:** Protein insufficiency can cause decreased muscular mass and strength. Adequate protein intake is necessary for muscle repair and growth.
- **Physical Activity:** Malnutrition can cause weariness and low energy levels, making it difficult for people to participate in physical activities that stimulate muscle development.

Cognitive Development

1. Brain Development:

- **Cognitive Function:** Iron, iodine, and omega-3 fatty acids are essential for brain development. Malnutrition can affect cognitive abilities like memory, concentration, and problem-solving ability.
- **Learning Difficulties:** Malnourished children may struggle to learn and succeed academically due to reduced brain function.

2. Behavioural Issues:

- **Mood and Behavior:** Nutrient shortages can impact neurotransmitter production, causing mood swings, irritation, and behavioral difficulties.

This can affect both social interactions and academic performance.

- **Attention and Focus:** Malnourished people may have difficulty paying attention and focusing, limiting their ability to learn and perform effectively in school or at work.

Immune System Function

1. Increased susceptibility to infections:

- **Weakened Immune Response:** Malnutrition weakens the immune system, rendering people more vulnerable to infections and diseases. This is related to a deficiency in critical nutrients needed for a strong immunological response.
- **Frequent Illness:** Malnourished people are more likely to suffer from frequent and severe diseases, which can impede growth and development.

2. Recovery from Illness:

- **Slow Recovery:** Malnutrition reduces the body's ability to fight infection and recover from disease. This can lead to longer recovery times and more serious health consequences.

Developmental Delays

1. Motor abilities:

- **Fine and Gross Motor Skills:** Malnutrition can hinder the development of fine and gross motor abilities. Children may struggle with activities that require coordination, balance, or strength.
- **Physical Activity:** Malnutrition might reduce a child's capacity to engage in physical play, which is essential for motor skill development.

2. Social and Emotional Development:

- **Social Interactions:** Malnourished children may struggle with social interactions owing to exhaustion, irritation, or behavioral concerns. This can affect their capacity to create and sustain connections.
- **Emotional Regulation:** Nutrient shortages can impair mood regulation, increasing the risk of anxiety and despair.

Long-term consequences

1. Chronic Health Conditions:

- **Lifelong Impact:** Malnutrition during critical growth phases might have long-term implications. Adults who were malnourished as children may be at a higher risk for chronic health issues like cardiovascular disease, diabetes, and osteoporosis.
- **Quality of Life:** Chronic health concerns caused by early malnutrition can have a substantial impact on an individual's quality of life, affecting their physical ability and general health.

2. Economic and social impact:

- **Educational attainment:** Poor cognitive and physical development can impair educational attainment, resulting in lower academic performance and fewer job chances.
- **Economic Productivity:** Malnutrition-related health conditions can impair a person's capacity to contribute economically, lowering their earning potential and overall productivity.

Addressing Malnutrition in ARFID

1. Early Intervention:

- **Timely Diagnosis:** Identifying and diagnosing ARFID early can prevent malnutrition and its consequences. Healthcare practitioners must be cautious in detecting indicators of ARFID and starting relevant therapies.
- **Comprehensive Treatment:** A multidisciplinary strategy involving healthcare specialists, such as dietitians, therapists, and physicians, is required to address both the nutritional and psychological elements of ARFID.

2. Nutritional Support:

- **Balanced Diet:** A balanced diet customized to individual needs can alleviate dietary deficits and promote growth and development.
- **Supplements:** If dietary adjustments are insufficient, supplements may be required to guarantee appropriate consumption of important nutrients. These should be taken with professional supervision.

3. Ongoing Monitoring:

- **Regular Checkups:** Continuous monitoring of growth and development is critical for altering treatment strategies and guaranteeing progression. Regular check-ups with healthcare experts can help track progress and identify potential concerns.

Long-Term Health Risks of ARFID

Avoidant/Restrictive Food Intake Disorder (ARFID) is a disorder that, if left untreated, can pose significant long-term health consequences. The restrictive eating practices associated with ARFID frequently lead to serious nutritional deficits and overall poor health. Understanding these hazards emphasizes the significance of early intervention and thorough care. The following are some of the long-term health hazards connected with ARFID:

Nutritional deficiencies and their consequences

1. Osteoporosis, Bone Health:

- **Calcium and Vitamin D Deficiency:** Inadequate calcium and vitamin D intake can cause weaker bones, increasing the risk of osteoporosis and fractures. This is especially concerning for people who get ARFID during their peak bone-building years in childhood and adolescence.
- **Long-Term Impact:** A shortage of these essential nutrients can lead to brittle bones and substantial mobility difficulties in adulthood.

2. Anemia:

- **Iron Deficiency:** Iron deficiency can result from a lack of iron-rich meals over time. This condition causes weariness, weakness, and reduced cognitive function.
- **Other Nutrient Deficiencies:** Vitamin B12 and folate deficiencies, which are also common in ARFID, can cause a variety of anemias and contribute to long-term health difficulties.

3. Protein-energy malnutrition:

- **Muscle Wasting:** Inadequate protein intake can cause muscle wasting and decreased muscular function, reducing overall physical strength and endurance.
- **Impaired Immune Function:** Protein is required for a healthy immune system. Long-term protein deficits can impair the immune system, rendering people more vulnerable to infections and diseases.

Growth and Development Issues

1. Stunted Growth:

- **Childhood Impact:** ARFID can cause stunted growth in children due to inadequate nutrient intake, limiting their height potential. This delayed growth can have lifelong consequences.
- **Delayed Puberty:** Nutritional inadequacies can cause puberty to be delayed, interfering with physical development and potentially leading to long-term hormonal imbalance.

2. Cognitive and Behavioural Development:

- **Brain Function:** Essential nutrients such as iron, omega-3 fatty acids, and vitamins support brain development and function. Deficiencies can result in reduced cognitive capacities, learning difficulties, and behavioral problems.
- **Mental Health:** Long-term malnutrition can lead to persistent mental health disorders including depression and anxiety, compounding the emotional and psychological difficulties that people with ARFID encounter.

Cardiovascular Health

1. Heart Disease:

- **Cholesterol and Lipid Levels:** Poor diet can cause abnormalities in cholesterol and lipid levels, raising the risk of heart disease. A diet low in essential fatty acids can exacerbate these difficulties.
- **Blood Pressure:** Nutritional deficits can disrupt blood pressure regulation, leading to hypertension and other cardiovascular issues.

2. Metabolic Syndrome:

- **Insulin Resistance:** Poor nutrition can lead to metabolic syndrome, which increases the risk of heart disease, stroke, and diabetes. Insulin resistance, a critical component of metabolic syndrome, can develop as a result of unhealthy eating habits.

Gastrointestinal Issues

1. Digestive Problems:

- **Gut Health:** Restrictive diets can disrupt gut bacteria, leading to digestive disorders like constipation, bloating, and IBS.
- **Gastrointestinal Disorders:** Long-term ARFID can raise the risk of developing gastrointestinal problems, such as gastritis and peptic ulcers, due to a lack of fiber and poor gut health.

2. Malabsorption:

- **Nutrient Absorption:** Prolonged malnutrition can hinder nutrient absorption, worsening deficiencies and creating a cycle of poor health.

Psychological and Social Impact

1. Chronic Mental Health Conditions:

- **Anxiety and Depression:** Restrictive eating can cause anxiety and despair, negatively impacting general well-being.
- **Social Isolation:** The social issues associated with ARFID, such as avoiding eating with others and feeling different or scrutinized, can result in long-term social isolation and loneliness.

2. Quality of Life:

- **Daily Functioning:** Nutritional inadequacies and health concerns can hinder everyday functioning and enjoyment of life. This can result in diminished productivity and a lower quality of life.
- **Relationships:** ARFID's psychological and emotional toll can affect relationships with family, friends, and lovers, resulting in social disengagement and isolation.

The Physical Toll of ARFID

Avoidant/Restrictive Food Intake Disorder (ARFID) can have a significant influence on both growth and development, particularly if it begins in childhood or adolescence. The restrictive eating behaviors associated with ARFID result in insufficient intake of key nutrients required for physical, cognitive, and emotional development.

Physical Growth

1.Stunted Growth:

- **Insufficient Nutrients:** Nutrient deficiency can cause stunted growth. Protein, vitamins, and minerals are all essential components for healthy growth. Children and adolescents with ARFID frequently ingest insufficient quantities of essential nutrients, resulting in stunted growth.
- **Height and Weight:** A lack of balanced nutrition can cause youngsters to be shorter and lighter than their peers, with long-term consequences for their entire physical development.

2. Delayed Puberty:

- **Nutritional Deficiencies:** Proper nutritional intake is crucial for hormonal changes that cause puberty. ARFID can delay puberty, resulting in delayed physical maturity and the possibility of long-term hormonal abnormalities.

3. Bone Health:

- **Calcium and Vitamin D Deficiency:** These nutrients promote bone growth and density. ARFID can cause weakened bones, increasing the risk of fractures and osteoporosis later in life.
- **Growth Plates:** Nutrient deficits can harm the growth plates in bones, which are important for bone lengthening. This can cause shorter stature and other bone abnormalities.

4. Muscle Development:

- **Protein Deficiency:** Protein is required for muscle growth and repair. Inadequate protein consumption can impair muscle mass and strength, limiting physical ability and endurance.
- **Physical Activity:** The weariness and low energy levels associated with malnutrition might impede participation in physical activities that are necessary for muscular growth.

Cognitive Development

1. Brain Development:

- **Critical Nutrients:** Iron, omega-3 fatty acids, and vitamins are essential for brain growth. Deficits in these nutrients can affect cognitive skills such as memory, attention, and problem-solving.
- **Learning Difficulties:** Children with ARFID may struggle academically due to diminished brain function and a decreased capacity to concentrate and learn.

2. Behavioural Issues:

- **Mood and Behavior:** Nutrient shortages can impact neurotransmitter production, causing mood swings, irritation, and behavioral difficulties. This can have an impact on social relationships and educational contexts.
- **Attention and Focus:** Malnourished youngsters may struggle with attention and focus, which can impede their academic achievement and social relationships.

Emotional and Social Development

1. Mental Health:

- **Anxiety and Depression:** Stress from a restricted diet and social obstacles can cause anxiety and despair. Nutrient shortages can also have a direct effect on mood regulation.
- **Emotional control:** Malnutrition can impair emotional control, making it difficult for people to cope with stress and keep their mood consistent.

2. Social Interactions:

- **Isolation:** Adolescents with ARFID may avoid food-related social events, resulting in isolation. This can stifle the growth of social skills and peer relationships.
- **Self-Esteem:** Struggling with eating disorders can influence self-esteem and body image, reducing general social confidence and the capacity to develop healthy connections.

Long-term consequences

1. Chronic Health Conditions:

- **Lifelong Impact:** Nutritional shortages throughout critical growth phases can result in chronic health conditions like osteoporosis, cardiovascular disease, and metabolic problems.
- **Quality of Life:** Chronic health problems caused by early malnutrition can have a substantial impact on a person's quality of life, affecting their physical ability and well-being.

2. Economic and social impact:

- **Educational attainment:** Poor cognitive and physical development can impair educational achievements, resulting in inferior academic attainment and fewer job possibilities.
- **Economic output:** Health concerns caused by ARFID might limit an individual's capacity to participate economically, lowering their earning potential and overall economic output.

The Increased Risk of Infections Due to Malnutrition

Malnutrition is a key issue in people with Avoidant/Restrictive Food Intake Disorder (ARFID), and one of the most serious effects is an increased risk of infection. The body's immune system is significantly reliant on enough diet to function correctly. When critical minerals are depleted, the immune system weakens, rendering people more vulnerable to illnesses. Here's a closer look at how malnutrition caused by ARFID increases the risk of infections:

The Role of Nutrition in Immune Function

1. Important Nutrients for Immune Function:

- **Proteins:** Proteins are the building components for antibodies and immune cells. Inadequate protein consumption can impair the immunological response, lowering the body's ability to combat infections.
- **Vitamins and Minerals:** Vitamins A, C, D, E, and B-complex, as well as minerals such as zinc, iron, and selenium, are essential for immunological function. Deficiencies in these nutrients can damage several components of the immune system.
- **Omega-3 Fatty Acids:** These fatty acids are anti-inflammatory and essential for immune cell function. A lack of omega-3s can result in an unbalanced immunological response.

2. Effects of Malnutrition on the Immune System:

- **Reduction in Immune Cells:** Malnutrition can reduce the quantity and function of immune cells such as T-cells, B-cells, and natural killer cells.
- **Impaired Antibody synthesis:** Nutrient shortages can interfere with the synthesis of antibodies, which are required for pathogen identification and neutralization.
- **Increased Inflammation:** Malnutrition can promote chronic inflammation, which weakens the immune system and impairs its ability to respond to infections.

Specific infections linked to malnutrition.

1. Respiratory Infections:

- **Common Cold and Influenza:** Malnutrition increases susceptibility to common respiratory illnesses, including colds and influenza. These infections may also continue longer and be more severe.

- **Pneumonia:** Malnourished people are more likely to have pneumonia, a deadly lung infection, due to reduced respiratory defenses and an impaired immune system.

2. Gastrointestinal Infections:

- **Gastroenteritis:** Inadequate nutrition can weaken the gut barrier, allowing microorganisms to cause gastroenteritis, resulting in diarrhea and vomiting.
- **Parasitic Infections:** Malnutrition can increase susceptibility to parasite illnesses including giardiasis and helminth infections, exacerbating nutritional inadequacies.

3. Skin Infections:

- **Dermatitis:** Vitamin and mineral deficiencies can impair skin integrity, increasing the risk of dermatitis and infections.
- **Wound Healing:** Malnutrition can slow wound healing, rendering people more susceptible to infections in cuts, scrapes, and surgical wounds.

4. Systemic Infections:

- **Sepsis:** Malnourished individuals are more likely to get sepsis, a potentially fatal illness caused by extensive inflammation in the body.

Mechanisms of Increased Infection Risk

1. Barrier Protection:

- **Skin and Mucosal Barriers:** Proper nutrition supports healthy skin and mucosal barriers, the first line of defense against infections. Malnutrition can break down these barriers, allowing pathogenic pathogens to enter more easily.

- **Gut Microbiota:** A well-balanced diet promotes a healthy gut microbiota, which is essential for fighting off gastrointestinal infections. Malnutrition can upset this balance, resulting in dysbiosis and increased infection risk.

2. Immune Cell Function:

- **Phagocyte Activity:** To properly engulf and eliminate infections, phagocytes require appropriate nutrition. Malnutrition can diminish activity and efficiency.
- **Cytokine creation:** Nutrients are required for the creation of cytokines, which are signaling molecules that control immune responses. Deficiencies can make the immune system less coordinated.

3. Antioxidant Defense:

- **Oxidative Stress:** Malnutrition can cause oxidative stress, damaging cells and tissues. Antioxidants such as vitamins C and E help to reduce this stress. Deficiencies in these nutrients can impair the body's ability to repair damage and resist illness.

Managing the Increased Infection Risk

1. Nutritional Rehabilitation:

- **Balanced Diet:** Eating a balanced diet with all important nutrients is crucial for improving immunological function. This comprises proteins, vitamins, minerals, and good fats.
- **Nutritional Supplements:** When food intake is insufficient, supplements may be required to rectify particular nutrient deficiencies under profes-

sional supervision.

2. Medical Monitoring:

- **Regular Health Check-Ups:** Regular monitoring by healthcare professionals can help detect and treat early indicators of malnutrition and illness.
- **Vaccinations:** Individuals with impaired immune systems may benefit from increased protection against common illnesses if they follow the recommended immunization schedule.

3. Hygiene and Infection Control:

- **Good hygiene practices:** Emphasising appropriate hygiene behaviors, such as frequent handwashing, can help lower the risk of illness.
- **Safe Food Handling:** Proper food handling and preparation can help to prevent foodborne infections, which are especially concerning for people with weakened immune systems.

Addressing Physical Consequences of ARFID with Medical Support

Addressing the physical effects of Avoidant/Restrictive Food Intake Disorder (ARFID) necessitates a collaborative and interdisciplinary approach including a variety of healthcare professionals. Early and adequate medical care is critical for reducing the negative effects of ARFID, which include malnutrition, growth delays, and general poor health.

Multidisciplinary Team Approach.

1. Paediatricians and Primary Care Physicians:

- **Initial Assessment and Diagnosis:** Pediatricians and primary care physicians are frequently the initial point of contact. They conduct extensive exams to diagnose ARFID, which include physical examinations, growth measurements, and nutritional evaluations.

- **Monitor Growth and Development:** Regular check-ups are critical for tracking growth patterns, weight, and developmental milestones. These professionals guarantee that any deviations from normal growth are identified and addressed promptly.

2. Registered Dietitians:

- **Nutritional Assessment:** Dietitians conduct thorough evaluations to discover deficiencies and dietary inadequacies. They build personalized food regimens to meet specific nutrient requirements.
- **Meal Planning and Education:** They teach patients and their families about balanced nutrition and assist in the creation of meal plans that cater to individual tastes and tolerances, thereby encouraging gradual dietary expansion.

3. Mental Health Professionals:

- **Therapy and Counselling:** Psychologists and therapists offer cognitive-behavioral therapy (CBT) and other treatments to address the psychological components of ARFID, including eating anxiety and anxieties.
- **Support for Families:** They provide assistance and support to families, assisting them in understanding ARFID and creating a supportive atmosphere.

Medical Intervention and Nutritional Support

1. Supplementation and fortification:

- **Vitamins and Minerals:** For severe deficiencies, multivitamins, iron, calcium, and vitamin D supplements may be prescribed to address imbalances.

- **High-Calorie Supplements:** For those who struggle to achieve their caloric demands through food alone, high-calorie nutritional supplements or shakes can be used to help them gain weight and improve their overall nutrition.

2. Medical Monitoring and Treatment:

- **Regular Blood Tests:** Regular blood tests assess nutrient levels, organ function, and overall health. This aids in the early detection and treatment of deficits.
- **Treatment of Complications:** Medical practitioners treat malnutrition-related consequences such as anemia, decreased immunological function, and delayed growth. This could include drugs or additional nutritional support.

3. Gastrointestinal Support:

- **Addressing Digestive Issues:** Many people with ARFID face digestive issues such as constipation, bloating, and acid reflux. To treat these symptoms, doctors may give drugs or recommend dietary changes.
- **Gut Health:** Dietitians may recommend probiotics or prebiotics to improve gut health and digestion, resulting in higher nutrient absorption.

Specialized Therapeutic Interventions

1. Feeding Therapy:

- **Occupational Therapists and Speech-Language Pathologists:** These specialists offer feeding therapy to help with sensory sensitivities, oral-motor skills, and swallowing challenges. Desensitization exercises and gradual exposure to novel textures and flavors are among the techniques used.

- **Behavioral Interventions:** Feeding therapists utilize behavioral tactics to promote healthy eating habits and alleviate eating-related anxiety.

2. Hospital-Based Programs:

- **Inpatient and Day Treatment Programmes:** Severe cases of ARFID may require intense treatment programs that include medical, nutritional, and psychological support in a structured setting.
- **Multidisciplinary Care:** These programs provide complete care from a team of professionals, ensuring that all aspects of ARFID are addressed concurrently.

Creating a supportive environment

1. Family Involvement:

- **Parental Guidance:** Educating parents about ARFID and including them in treatment strategies is vital. Parents are taught how to prepare nutritious meals, deal with mealtime issues, and encourage their child's development.
- **Creating a Positive Eating Environment:** Families are advised to make mealtimes stress-free and enjoyable since this can help reduce anxiety and promote healthy eating habits.

2. School Support:

- **Collaboration with Schools:** Medical practitioners collaborate with schools to provide children's dietary needs during the school day. This can involve providing suitable snacks, meals, and accommodations for those who have difficulty eating.

- **Education and Awareness:** Increasing ARFID awareness among teachers and school staff fosters a supportive environment while reducing any stigma or misunderstandings.

Debunking Myths: Understanding the Complexities of Nutrition in ARFID

One prevalent myth concerning Avoidant/Restrictive Food Intake disease (ARFID) is that people with the disease do not want to eat. This myth might cause misunderstandings and a lack of empathy for persons dealing with ARFID. In actuality, the problem is significantly more complex, stemming from specific anxieties, sensory sensitivities, and a lack of interest in food rather than a mere dislike for eating.

The Complex Nature of ARFID

1. Sensory sensitivities:

- **Texture and Taste Aversions:** Many people with ARFID have heightened sensory sensitivities, which make certain textures, tastes, or scents of food overwhelming and unpleasant. This can result in a relatively limited diet since they avoid foods that cause unpleasant sensory impressions.
- **Worry of Negative Sensory Experiences:** The worry of meeting an unpleasant texture or flavor can generate significant anxiety during mealtimes, decreasing people's willingness to try new foods.

2. Fear-Based Avoidance:

- **Fear of Choking:** ARFID patients may suffer fear of choking or vomiting as a result of a painful incident in the past. This fear might be so strong that individuals avoid foods believed to be harmful, even if they previously enjoyed them.

- **Fear of Gastrointestinal Distress:** Worrying about stomach pain, nausea, or other gastrointestinal problems can lead to restrictive eating habits.

3. Lack of Interest in Food:

- **Low Appetite:** In contrast to other eating disorders that restrict food intake owing to body image issues, persons with ARFID may simply lack an appetite. This could be related to a low appetite in general or a lack of inner motivation to eat.
- **Monotony and predictability:** Some people find comfort in eating the same items repeatedly. The predictability of these "safe" foods relieves anxiety while limiting dietary variety and nutritional adequacy.

Addressing the Myth: Empathy and Understanding

1. Recognise the Challenges:

- **Empathizing with Sensory Issues:** Recognising that sensory sensitivities can make eating a difficult experience is critical. It is not a lack of desire to eat, but rather an excessive response to specific sensory inputs.
- **Acknowledging fears:** Recognising that fears of choking or gastrointestinal upset are real and deeply engrained can help you address the situation with compassion.

2. Creating a Supportive Environment:

- **Safe and comfortable dining areas:** Ensuring that mealtime conditions are quiet and stress-free can help reduce anxiety and make eating more enjoyable.
- **Gradual Exposure to New Foods:** Introducing new foods slowly and in tiny amounts, combined with positive reinforcement, can help people with ARFID broaden their dietary options without feeling overwhelmed.

3. Professional Intervention:

- **Therapy and counselling:** Cognitive-behavioral therapy (CBT) and other treatments can assist people in overcoming underlying worries and anxiety about eating. Therapists can help individuals create coping techniques and ultimately desensitize them to frightened meals.
- **Nutritional Support:** Working with a trained dietitian can help ensure that people with ARFID get enough nourishment. Dietitians can design meal regimens that provide a variety of nutrients while accommodating sensory and fear-based restrictions.

Myth: There's a "Cure" for ARFID

One common myth concerning Avoidant/Restrictive Food Intake Disorder (ARFID) is that there is a simple "cure" for the disorder. This misperception can lead to unreasonable expectations and dissatisfaction among ARFID patients and their families. Understanding that ARFID is a complex, varied illness that necessitates continuing management rather than a single cure is critical for effective therapy and support.

Understanding ARFID as a chronic condition.

1. The nature of ARFID:

- **Chronic and evolving:** ARFID is frequently a chronic disorder that can last into adulthood if not treated properly. It entails maintaining restrictive eating habits due to sensory sensitivity, fear of undesirable repercussions, or a lack of interest in food.
- **Individual Variability:** The presentation of ARFID might differ significantly between individuals. What helps for one person may not work for another, and symptoms can fluctuate over time.

2. Treatment Focus:

- **Management Over Cure:** The goal of ARFID treatment is to manage symptoms effectively, improve nutritional intake, and enhance the quality of life. This approach focuses on gradual progress rather than a definitive cure.
- **Multi-Disciplinary Approach:** Effective management typically involves a team of healthcare professionals, including therapists, dietitians, and physicians, working together to address the various aspects of the disorder.

Comprehensive Treatment Strategies

1. Therapy and Psychological Support:

- **Cognitive-behavioral therapy (CBT):** CBT is one of the most effective treatment options for ARFID. It assists individuals in identifying and challenging negative attitudes and behaviors associated with food and eating, progressively lowering anxiety and avoidance.
- **Exposure Therapy:** This strategy involves gradual, controlled exposure to feared foods or eating settings, which helps people gain tolerance and diminish their fear responses over time.

2. Nutritional Intervention:

- **Personalized Meal Plans:** Registered dietitians create meal plans tailored to individuals' nutritional needs, sensory preferences, and food aversions. These plans intend to introduce variation gradually.
- **Supplementation:** In circumstances where nutritional intake is considerably compromised, dietary supplements may be required to guarantee optimal nutrient levels.

3. Medical Monitoring:

- **Regular Health Check-Ups:** Regular check-ups assess growth, weight, and overall health, allowing for rapid adjustments to treatment strategies.
- **Addressing Medical Complications:** Healthcare providers handle any physical health difficulties caused by ARFID, such as nutrient deficits or gastrointestinal disorders.

4. Creating a Supportive Environment:

- **Family Education and Involvement:** Educating and integrating families in ARFID treatment helps foster a supportive home environment. Family members learn how to promote healthy eating habits without imposing pressure or stress.
- **School and Community Support:** Working with schools and community resources ensures that people with ARFID receive assistance in a variety of settings, including academic and social.

Shifting Perspectives: From Cure to Management

1. Realistic Expectations:

- **Progress Over Perfection:** Emphasizing minor, gradual improvements over a total "cure" can boost motivation and prevent frustration.
- **Ongoing Effort:** Managing ARFID necessitates consistent effort and flexibility. Recognizing setbacks as a regular part of the process might help individuals and families stick to long-term treatment plans.

2. Celebrating Milestones:

- **Acknowledging Achievements:** Celebrating little wins, like trying a new food or lowering anxiety during mealtimes, reinforces positive development and encourages continuing efforts.

- **Maintaining Motivation:** Regularly reflecting on progress and creating reasonable goals will help retain motivation and a positive view on the journey towards better-managing ARFID.

The Importance of Individualized Nutritional Needs

When it comes to treating Avoidant/Restrictive Food Intake Disorder (ARFID), one size does not fit all. Each individual with ARFID faces distinct issues, preferences, and nutritional needs. Tailoring dietary assistance to these specific demands is critical for optimal management and general well-being.

Understanding the Need for Individualization.

1. Diverse ARFID Presentations:

- **Various Symptoms:** ARFID manifests itself in a variety of ways, including sensory aversions, a fear of choking, and a general disinterest in eating. Because of the variety of symptoms, nutritional methods must be tailored to each individual's unique needs.
- **Personal Preferences and Tolerances:** A person with ARFID may be able to tolerate meals that another person cannot. Personal tastes and sensory tolerances are important considerations when deciding on an ideal diet.

2. Nutritional deficiencies and health risks:

- **Identifying Deficiencies:** People with ARFID are at risk for a variety of dietary deficiencies due to their restricted diets. A thorough nutritional assessment is required to identify and correct these deficiencies.
- **Tailored Supplementation:** Supplements may be required to treat certain deficiencies, but the type and quantity required will differ for each individual.

Steps to Developing an Individualized Nutritional Plan

1. Comprehensive Nutritional Assessment:

- **Initial Evaluation:** A registered dietitian conducts a detailed assessment of the individual's dietary habits, nutrient intake, and health status. This includes reviewing food diaries, conducting interviews, and possibly performing lab tests to identify deficiencies.
- **Personalized Analysis:** Understanding the individual's dietary preferences, aversions, and eating patterns aids in developing a nutritionally appropriate and acceptable strategy for the person with ARFID.

2. Creating a Tailored Meal Plan:

- **Balancing Nutrition and Preferences:** The meal plan should include meals that the individual can tolerate while also providing a balanced intake of vital nutrients. This could entail identifying alternative sources of nutrients from approved meals.
- **Gradual Introduction of New Foods:** New foods should be introduced gradually and carefully, utilizing tactics like matching with safe meals or positive reinforcement to foster adoption.

3. Ongoing Monitoring and Adjustment:

- **Regular follow-ups:** Continuous monitoring and regular follow-up sessions with the dietician are essential for tracking progress, making appropriate changes, and addressing any emergent concerns.
- **Adaptability:** The nutritional plan should be flexible enough to accommodate changing needs, preferences, and progress. Adjustments may be required to reflect increased food variety and tolerance.

The Role of Family and Support Systems

1. Educating Families:

- **Understanding Nutritional Needs:** Families play a crucial role in assisting individuals with ARFID. Educating them on the value of individualized nutrition allows them to comprehend and support the dietary plan.
- **Creating a Supportive Environment:** Families can assist by cooking meals that are consistent with the nutritional plan, fostering happy eating experiences, and avoiding pressure or unfavorable remarks about food choices.

2. Collaboration with Healthcare Providers:

- **Multidisciplinary Approach:** Working with a team of healthcare providers, such as therapists, pediatricians, and gastroenterologists, ensures a comprehensive approach to addressing ARFID. This partnership helps to address both the physical and psychological aspects of the illness.
- **Coordinated Care:** Regular communication between the dietitian and other healthcare practitioners ensures that the nutritional plan is effectively integrated into the overall treatment strategy.

Long-Term Advantages of Individualised Nutrition

1. Improved Nutritional Status:

- **Addressing Deficiencies:** Tailored nutritional regimens assist in addressing deficiencies and ensure that the individual gets enough nutrients for growth, development, and overall health.
- **Enhanced Growth and Development:** Individualised nutrition is critical for appropriate growth and development in children with ARFID, allowing

them to reach their full potential.

2. Improved Quality of Life:

- **Reduced Anxiety Around Food:** Respecting individuals' dietary preferences and demands might lead to less anxiety during mealtimes.
- **Increased Food range:** Over time, a personalized approach can help people broaden their diet, increasing the range of foods they can eat and improving their general connection with food.

3. Empowerment and Autonomy:

- **Building Confidence:** Involving individuals in the planning process and honoring their preferences can boost confidence and give them control over their eating habits.
- **Encouraging Independence:** As people learn to manage their dietary demands, they gain independence and are more equipped to make good food choices.

4

Chapter 4: The Emotional and Social Impact of ARFID

The Emotional Burden of ARFID

Avoidant/Restrictive Food Intake Disorder (ARFID) involves more than just food aversions or restricted eating; it is frequently associated with major psychological issues, notably anxiety disorders. Understanding the complex association between ARFID and anxiety is critical to delivering comprehensive care and successful treatment techniques.

Understanding the Connection

1. Shared Underlying Factors:

- **Sensory sensitivities:** Many people with ARFID have increased sensory sensitivity, making specific textures, tastes, and food scents unpleasant. These sensory sensitivities are frequently associated with anxiety, as the anticipation of unfavorable sensory experiences can cause severe distress.
- **Fear-Based Avoidance:** Anxiety disorders are defined by excessive fear

and avoidance behaviours. In ARFID, these anxieties frequently emerge as a fear of choking, vomiting, or feeling gastrointestinal distress, resulting in restrictive eating habits.

2. Effects of Anxiety on Eating Behaviours:

- **Increased Arousal and Vigilance:** Anxiety can increase alertness and attentiveness, making people more aware of potential food-related risks. This heightened condition may worsen eating-related concerns and avoidance behaviours.
- **Conditioned Responses:** Anxiety can cause conditioned reactions, in which previous negative experiences with eating (such as choking or gagging) reinforce avoidance behaviours. These conditioned reflexes might be difficult to overcome without specific intervention.

Anxiety Disorders Commonly Associated with ARFID.

1. General Anxiety Disorder (GAD):

- **Excessive worry:** Individuals with GAD have a persistent and excessive concern about many aspects of their lives, including food and eating. This anxiety can lead to restrictive eating habits and fear-based avoidance of particular foods.

2. Social Anxiety Disorder:

- **Fear of Judgment:** Social anxiety disorder is characterized by acute dread of being judged or embarrassed in social circumstances. This can impact eating habits, as people may avoid eating in public or social situations for fear of being judged negatively.
- **Isolation:** Avoiding social meals can lead to isolation and worsen restrictive eating habits.

3. Obsessive-Compulsive Disorder (OCD):

- **Obsessive Thoughts and Compulsions:** Obsessive concerns about contamination, food safety, or fear of choking can lead to compulsive behaviors like frequent checking, food avoidance, or ritualistic eating.
- **Rigid Eating Rules:** The desire for control and certainty can lead to strict eating habits and a severely restricted diet.

4. Post-Traumatic Stress Disorder (PTSD):

- **Traumatic Experiences:** Traumatic encounters with food, such as choking, severe allergic responses, or food poisoning, can trigger PTSD. The trauma may cause acute anxiety and avoidance of certain foods or eating settings.

Managing Anxiety during ARFID Treatment

1. Comprehensive assessment:

- **Identifying coexisting anxiety disorders:** A thorough assessment by a mental health practitioner can aid in identifying coexisting anxiety disorders and their impact on eating habits.
- **Tailored Treatment Approach:** Understanding the precise type and severity of anxiety can help guide a treatment approach that targets both the anxiety and the restrictive eating patterns associated with ARFID.

2. Integrated Therapeutic Approaches:

- **Cognitive-behavioral therapy (CBT):** CBT can effectively treat anxiety disorders and ARFID. It assists individuals in identifying and challenging negative thoughts and behaviours, developing coping mechanisms, and ultimately decreasing avoidance behaviours.
- **Exposure Therapy:** Gradual exposure to feared meals or eating settings,

combined with relaxation techniques, can help alleviate anxiety and increase tolerance to previously avoided foods.

3. Mindfulness and relaxation techniques:

- **Mindfulness Practices:** Mindfulness methods can help people stay present and lessen worry over eating. Mindful eating promotes a nonjudgmental awareness of food and eating experiences.
- **Relaxation Techniques:** Deep breathing, progressive muscle relaxation, and visualization can all help you control your anxiety and feel more peaceful during meals.

4. Supportive Environment:

- **Family Involvement:** Educating and enrolling family members in treatment can provide crucial assistance. Families may help to promote a stress-free, supportive eating environment and maintain excellent eating habits.
- **Support Groups:** Connecting with others who have gone through similar situations through support groups or online communities can help you feel less isolated and more encouraged.

Feeling Isolated and Alone Due to ARFID

Living with Avoidant/Restrictive Food Intake Disorder (ARFID) can be very isolated. The particular obstacles associated with ARFID, such as limited food options, eating anxiety, and social stigma, frequently result in feelings of isolation and loneliness. Understanding these emotional effects and developing strategies to treat them is critical for the well-being of people with ARFID.

Sources of Isolation

1. Social avoidance:

- **Avoiding Social Events:** Many social activities and gatherings center on food. Individuals with ARFID may avoid settings involving unusual foods or eating in front of others.
- **Feeling Out of Place:** Even when they attend social activities, people with ARFID may feel out of place or unusual because of their restrictive eating habits. This feeling of not fitting in can further deter social participation.

2. Misunderstanding:

- **Misunderstanding by Others:** Others may misinterpret ARFID as finicky eating or lack of willpower. This misconception might lead to judgmental comments or unwanted advice, leaving people with ARFID feeling misunderstood and alienated.
- **Difficulty Explaining ARFID:** The disorder's complexity and the intimate nature of food-related issues make it difficult to express what people are going through, which leads to feelings of isolation.

3. Emotional Toll:

- **Anxiety and Depression:** ARFID can cause anxiety and melancholy, leading to feelings of isolation. The continual preoccupation with food and eating might take over their thoughts, leaving little room for social connections.
- **Shame and Embarrassment:** Feeling guilty or embarrassed about their eating habits might cause people with ARFID to hide their problems from others, exacerbating their isolation.

Strategies for Overcoming Isolation.

1. Creating a Support System:

- **Educating Family and Friends:** Educating loved ones about ARFID helps increase understanding and support. When loved ones understand the challenges of ARFID, they can offer more emotional support and foster a more tolerant environment.
- **Open conversation:** Encouraging open and honest conversation about one's needs and feelings can make people with ARFID feel more connected and understood. Sharing their stories can alleviate the effects of isolation.

2. Support Groups:

- **Support Groups:** Joining support groups for those with ARFID helps foster a sense of camaraderie and understanding. These organizations provide a secure environment in which to discuss experiences, problems, and accomplishments with others who encounter similar difficulties.
- **Online Communities:** ARFID-specific forums and social media groups can be useful resources for connecting and supporting one another. These platforms enable people to reach out and connect with others from all around the world who understand their path.

3. Engaging in Non-Food-Centric Activities:

- **Finding Alternative Social Activities:** Finding other social activities can assist those with ARFID retain social relationships without the stress of eating. Hiking, arts & crafts, and going to the movies are all fun ways to socialize.
- **Recommending Alternative Venues:** When planning social events, recommending venues or activities that are not food-related can make socializing more enjoyable. This can help people with ARFID feel involved

without the added stress of dealing with food.

4. Professional Support:

- **Therapy:** Working with a therapist who specializes in eating disorders can help address the emotional impact of ARFID. Therapy can help you manage anxiety, reduce shame, and improve your social connections.
- **Counseling:** Counselling sessions can assist individuals in exploring their feelings of loneliness and developing coping methods to handle these emotions. A counselor can offer a safe place to work through the emotional difficulties linked with ARFID.

5. Practice Self-Compassion:

- **Positive self-talk:** Encourage positive self-talk and self-compassion to help people with ARFID overcome feelings of isolation. Reminding oneself that their troubles are valid and that they are not alone can help them feel better emotionally.
- **Celebrating small victories:** Recognising and applauding minor accomplishments, such as trying a new dish or attending a social gathering, can increase confidence and lessen feelings of loneliness.

The Risk of Depression in Individuals with ARFID

Avoidant/Restrictive dietary Intake Disorder (ARFID) is more than just a dietary issue; it can also cause major psychological problems, including an increased risk of depression. Understanding the link between ARFID and depression is critical for delivering comprehensive care and assisting people on their path to recovery.

The Link Between ARFID and Depression

1. Emotional strain:

- **chronic stress:** The everyday stress of regulating food intake, dealing with eating anxiety, and dealing with the physical implications of ARFID can all lead to long-term emotional distress. This constant tension can strain a person's mental health over time, leading to depression.
- **Emotions of despondency:** The ongoing problems and disappointments connected with ARFID might cause emotions of despondency. When people believe they are unable to overcome their eating disorders, it has a detrimental impact on their attitude and view on life.

2. Social Isolation:

- **Avoidance of Social Situations:** Avoiding food-related social events can cause severe isolation. Missing out on social connections and feeling cut off from peers can exacerbate feelings of loneliness and melancholy.
- **Lack of Understanding:** Misunderstandings and judgments regarding ARFID by others can make people feel alienated and ignored, worsening depression.

3. Impact on Self-Esteem:

- **Body Image Issues:** ARFID may hurt body image and self-esteem. Concerns about growth, development, and physical attractiveness caused by malnutrition can result in low self-esteem, which is a risk factor for depression.
- **Sense of Failure:** Struggling with eating and feeling different from others can result in feelings of failure or inadequacy. This unfavorable self-perception may contribute to depression symptoms.

Recognizing Symptoms of Depression in ARFID Patients

1. Mood changes:

- **Persistent sadness:** Persistent sensations of sadness, emptiness, or hopelessness are strong signs of depression. These feelings may be present for most of the day, or almost every day.
- **Irritation:** Depression, especially in children and adolescents, can cause irritation, impatience, or aggression.

2. Behavioural Changes:

- **Loss of Interest:** A noteworthy loss in interest or pleasure in previously appreciated activities may indicate depression.
- **Social retreat:** Isolation and retreat from friends, family, and social activities may suggest depression symptoms.

3. Physical Symptoms:

- **Fatigue:** Persistent exhaustion or low energy levels, especially without physical exercise, may indicate depression.
- **Sleep Disturbances:** Depression can disrupt sleep habits, resulting in insomnia or excessive sleeping.

4. Cognitive Symptoms:

- **Difficulty Concentrating:** Depression can impair cognitive function, causing difficulties with concentration, decision-making, and memory.
- **Negative Thoughts:** Depression is associated with frequent negative thoughts, such as feelings of worthlessness, remorse, and self-criticism.

Managing Depression in ARFID Patients

1. Professional Support:

- **Therapy:** Cognitive Behavioural Therapy (CBT) is useful for treating both depression and ARFID. It enables people to identify and fight negative thought patterns, create coping mechanisms, and enhance their mood.
- **Medication: In** some circumstances, medication may be administered to alleviate depression symptoms. Antidepressants can boost mood and overall mental health.

2. Integrated Treatment Approach:

- **Collaborative therapy:** A multidisciplinary team of therapists, dietitians, and medical specialists can offer comprehensive therapy. This guarantees that the psychological and nutritional needs of people with ARFID are met.
- **Holistic Interventions:** Incorporating holistic interventions, such as mindfulness practices, relaxation techniques, and stress management tactics, can help to improve overall mental health and well-being.

3. Establishing an assistance Network:

- **Family and Friends:** Educating family and friends about the danger of depression in individuals with ARFID can improve their ability to provide effective assistance. Encourage open communication and understanding to lessen feelings of isolation.
- **Support Groups:** Attending support groups, whether in person or online, can provide a sense of belonging and understanding. Connecting with others who are facing similar issues can provide emotional support and alleviate feelings of loneliness.

4. Promoting Self-Care and Resilience:

- **Self-Compassion:** Practicing self-compassion and positive self-talk can aid in managing depression symptoms. Focusing on qualities and accomplishments, no matter how minor, can increase self-esteem.
- **Healthy Lifestyle:** Promoting a healthy lifestyle, which includes frequent physical activity, enough sleep, and a well-balanced diet, can benefit overall mental health. Participating in fun activities and hobbies can help boost mood and reduce stress.

The Social Impact of ARFID

Living with Avoidant/Restrictive Food Intake Disorder (ARFID) frequently involves dealing with misunderstandings and judgments from others. A lack of awareness regarding ARFID can result in cruel comments and social stigma, affecting an individual's emotional well-being. Learning to deal with unfavorable comments and judgments is essential for developing resilience and sustaining self-esteem.

Understanding the Source of Negative Comments.

1. Lack of Awareness:

- **Misconceptions:** ARFID is often misunderstood as fussy eating or a lack of willpower. This lack of comprehension can result in rude or dismissive responses.
- **Ignorance:** People may underestimate the intricacy and gravity of ARFID, believing it is something that can be easily addressed with more effort or determination.

2. Societal Pressures:

- **Diet Culture:** Society's emphasis on ideal eating behaviors and body images can lead to the judgement of those who do not conform to these norms. People with ARFID may experience scrutiny since their eating habits do not meet societal norms.

- **Fear of Difference:** Differences in behavior, such as unusual eating patterns, might make others uncomfortable, prompting harsh comments as a coping mechanism.

Strategies for Handling Negative Comments

1. Educating Others:

- **Informative Responses:** When confronted with harsh comments, a simple explanation of ARFID can assist educate the person and prevent future misunderstandings. For example, mentioning, "ARFID is a recognized eating disorder that involves severe food aversions and isn't just picky eating," can help to clarify.
- **Sharing Resources:** Providing others with resources or informational materials concerning ARFID can also assist raise awareness and comprehension.

2. Setting Boundaries:

- **Assertive Communication:** Clarify and assert your boundaries. You can respond, "I understand your concerns, but comments regarding my eating habits are not helpful. I'm working on it with my healthcare team."
- **Limiting Exposure:** If specific people continue to make harmful comments despite your attempts to educate them, you may need to limit your interactions with them to preserve your mental health.

3. Create a Supportive Network:

- **Supportive Friends and Family:** Surround yourself with those who understand and support you. Having a network of sympathetic and knowledgeable people can provide emotional support and help balance out unfavorable interactions.

- **Support Groups:** Joining a support group, whether in person or online, can help you connect with others who have had similar experiences. Sharing your challenges and coping skills with those who understand can be empowering.

4. Practicing Self-Compassion:

- **Positive Self-Talk:** Challenge negative thoughts with positive affirmations about yourself and your journey. Remind yourself that ARFID is a medical problem that does not represent your personality or willpower.
- **Focus on Progress:** Recognise and appreciate your progress, no matter how tiny. Recognizing your accomplishments can improve your self-esteem and resilience.

Coping With Internalised Judgements

1. Identifying Negative Thoughts:

- **Self-awareness:** Recognise negative ideas or beliefs influenced by others' opinions. Recognize that these thoughts are external judgments, not realities about oneself.
- **Journaling:** Writing down your thoughts and feelings can help you process and challenge unpleasant internalized beliefs. Think about the sources of these thoughts and if they are based on facts or misconceptions.

2. Reframing Negative Thoughts:

- **Using Cognitive Restructuring:** Use cognitive-behavioral therapy to reframe negative thinking. For example, if you believe that "I should be able to eat like everyone else," reframe it as "I'm taking steps to improve my eating habits at my own pace."

- **Focusing on Strengths:** Change your focus from perceived flaws to your strengths and abilities. Remind yourself of your tenacity and the strides you've made in managing ARFID.

3. Seeking Professional Support:

- **Therapy:** Working with a therapist might help you build techniques for dealing with unfavorable comments and judgments. Therapy can also provide a secure environment in which to confront and question internalized negative beliefs.
- **Counseling:** Individual or group counseling can provide extra support and advice. Counselors can help you develop confidence and resilience in the face of both external and internal criticism.

Missing Out on Social Events and Activities Due to ARFID

Avoidant/Restrictive Food Intake Disorder (ARFID) has a substantial impact on both an individual's physical health and eating habits, as well as their social life. Food-related anxiety and restrictions can cause people to miss out on crucial social gatherings and activities, contributing to feelings of loneliness and isolation. Understanding the impact of ARFID on social relationships and overcoming these obstacles is critical for leading a successful social life.

The Social Impact of ARFID

1. Anxiety during food-related events:

- **Fear of judgment:** Food plays an important role in many social occasions, including parties, dinners, and holiday celebrations. For those with ARFID, the anxiety of being scrutinized for their eating habits can prompt them to avoid these activities entirely.

- **Strange meals:** The appearance of strange meals, or the pressure to try new cuisines, can cause anxiety. This dread can make social gatherings difficult rather than joyful, prompting people to decline invites.

2. Feeling out of place:

- **Social norms:** Eating is frequently viewed as a social activity, and variations from standard eating habits can make people with ARFID feel out of place or self-conscious. This can cause reluctance to participate in group activities.
- **Questions & Comments:** Constant questioning or comments regarding eating habits from others can be burdensome and make people feel uneasy. This may deter them from attending social events.

3. Emotional Toll:

- **Loneliness:** Missing out on social gatherings can cause emotions of loneliness and isolation from friends and family. The urge to avoid food-related stress might cause severe social isolation.
- **Relationship Impact:** Declining social invitations regularly might strain relationships because friends and relatives may not understand why you are avoiding them. This might lead to misconceptions and a reduction in social support.

Strategies for navigating social situations

1. Planning Ahead:

- **Communicating Needs:** Before attending an event, communicate your needs with the host. Informing them of your dietary limitations will allow them to better accommodate you and lessen your concern about the available food selections.

- **Bringing Safe Foods:** If feasible, please bring your safe foods to the event. This guarantees that you have something to eat comfortably while also reducing the burden of seeking suitable selections.

2. Engage in non-food activities:

- **Engaging in Activities:** Concentrate on the non-food parts of the event, such as discussions, games, or other activities. Shifting your emphasis away from food can allow you to enjoy social interactions without feeling stressed.
- **Suggesting Alternative Gatherings:** Plan social activities that do not revolve around food, such as going to the movies, hiking, or attending a cultural event. This enables you to engage in social situations without the anxiety associated with eating.

3. Creating a Supportive Social Network:

- **Educating Friends and Family:** Educate close friends and relatives about ARFID to better understand your issues. Having a supportive social network that understands your requirements can help you manage social occasions more effectively.
- **Finding Understanding Peers:** Look for people or groups who understand and support your condition. Being with people who understand your position can alleviate stress and make social interactions more enjoyable.

4. Practice Coping Strategies:

- **Mindfulness and Relaxation:** Use mindfulness and relaxation practices to reduce anxiety before and during social gatherings. Deep breathing, meditation, and gradual muscular relaxation can all help you stay calm.
- **Positive Self-Talk:** Remind yourself that it is acceptable to have varied eating patterns and that your worth is not defined by what or how you eat. Remind yourself that your presence and participation are important.

5. Seeking Professional Support:

- **Therapy:** Working with a therapist can assist you in developing techniques for managing social anxiety associated with ARFID. Cognitive-behavioral therapy (CBT) is especially successful in treating the cognitive patterns and behaviors related to social avoidance.
- **Counseling:** Group counseling or support groups can foster a sense of belonging and mutual understanding. Connecting with people who have similar issues can provide both practical guidance and emotional support.

Difficulties with Relationships and Dating

Living with Avoidant/Restrictive Food Intake Disorder (ARFID) can present considerable obstacles in terms of relationships and dating. The disorder's effects on eating habits and social interactions can cause misunderstandings, anxiety, and difficulties in building and maintaining close relationships. Individuals with ARFID, on the other hand, can overcome these challenges and form meaningful connections with the help of communication, understanding, and support.

Challenges in Relationships and Dating

1. Fear of Judgement and Misunderstanding:

- **Explaining ARFID:** Explaining ARFID to a possible spouse can be challenging. There is a common anxiety that others would not understand or will criticize you based on your eating habits.
- **Misconceptions:** Many individuals may associate ARFID with regular picky eating or assume it is easily overcome, resulting in a lack of empathy or support.

2. Anxiety about food-related activities:

- **Eating Out:** Dating frequently includes food-related activities such as dining out, which can be unpleasant for those with ARFID. The pressure to consume things that cause anxiety can make these outings less enjoyable.
- **Social Events:** Attending social gatherings with a spouse can be difficult because they often entail food. Navigating these situations can be extremely stressful and anxiety-inducing.

3. Impact on Intimacy and Trust:

- **Emotional Vulnerability:** ARFID may cause feelings of guilt or embarrassment over eating behaviors. Being open and genuine about these problems can be challenging, affecting emotional intimacy.
- **Trust Issues:** If your partner does not fully understand or support your condition, it can cause trust issues and strain on the relationship.

Strategies for Managing Relationship Challenges

1.Open and Honest Communication:

- **Early Conversations:** Establish open and honest communication regarding ARFID early in the relationship. Explaining your disease and how it affects your everyday life can assist to create realistic expectations and build understanding.
- **Setting Boundaries:** Be clear about your boundaries and comfort levels in food and social situations. Letting your partner know what causes your anxiety and what makes you feel safe will help them assist you more effectively.

2. Educating Your Partner:

- **Provide Information:** Share ARFID-related resources and information with your partner. Helping them comprehend the nuances of the disease might boost their empathy and support.

- **Encourage Involvement:** If your partner is willing, invite them to attend therapy sessions or support groups with you. This can give them a better grasp of your problems and how to help.

3. Find Alternative Activities:

- **Plan non-food-centered dates:** Hiking, visiting museums, and going to the movies can all be relaxing and pleasurable activities.
- **Cooking Together:** If you feel at ease, making meals together can be a great way to share your safe foods with your partner while also connecting.

4. Building Trust and Intimacy:

- **Gradual Disclosure:** Share your experiences and challenges with ARFID gradually, allowing trust and closeness to develop over time. Being patient with both yourself and your partner is essential.
- **Fostering Emotional Support:** Encourage open dialogue about feelings and emotions. A helpful partner would want to understand and assist you overcome your difficulties.

5. Seeking Professional Support:

- **Couples Therapy:** Couples therapy offers a safe area to address how ARFID affects your relationship. A therapist can work with both partners to establish communication and support techniques.
- **Individual treatment:** Continuing individual treatment will help you handle the emotional and psychological components of ARFID, ultimately improving your relationship.

6. Practice Self-Compassion:

- **Recognise Your Efforts:** Recognize and appreciate the work you are doing to manage your health and your relationship. Self-compassion can help alleviate emotions of guilt and inadequacy.

- **Positive Affirmations:** Remind yourself that you are worthy of love and care, regardless of your dietary habits. Positive self-talk can help you gain confidence and self-esteem.

Building Resilience: Empowering Yourself and Your Loved Ones

Managing Avoidant/Restrictive Food Intake Disorder (ARFID) entails not only addressing the eating behaviors but also dealing with the resulting anxiety and emotional difficulties. Developing appropriate coping techniques can have a major impact on emotional well-being and general quality of life. Here are some ways of dealing with ARFID-related anxiety and emotions.

Understanding the Emotional Impact of ARFID

1. Recognising Anxiety Triggers:

- **Food-related anxiety:** Fear of new foods, textures, and eating in public can cause intense anxiety.
- **Social Situations:** Food-related incidents can cause stress and feelings of isolation.

2. Emotional Responses:

- **humiliation and Embarrassment:** Feeling different or condemned based on eating habits might result in humiliation.
- **Dissatisfaction and Hopelessness:** Struggling with food intake can lead to dissatisfaction and a lack of optimism for recovery.

Coping Strategies for Anxiety and Emotions

1. Mindfulness and relaxation techniques:

- **Mindful Practices:** Mindfulness exercises, such as meditation and mindful eating, can assist in alleviating anxiety. These practices entail focusing on the present moment and monitoring thoughts and emotions without judgment.
- **Breathing Exercises:** Deep breathing exercises, such as diaphragmatic breathing or box breathing, can help to relax the nervous system and reduce anxiety. Using these tactics daily can help you handle stress in difficult situations.

2. Cognitive-Behavioral Techniques:

- **Challenging Negative Thoughts:** Recognise and combat negative thoughts about food and self-worth. Replace them with more balanced, good thoughts. For example, if you believe that "I can't eat like everyone else," reframe it as "I'm working on improving my eating habits at my own pace."
- **Exposure Therapy:** Gradual exposure to feared foods or eating settings might help alleviate anxiety over time. Begin with modest, manageable steps, gradually increasing the level of difficulty as you gain familiarity.

3. Build a Support System:

- **Connecting with Others:** Connect with others through support groups or forums to exchange experiences and coping skills with those who understand ARFID. Connecting with others who are facing similar issues can provide emotional support and minimize feelings of isolation.
- **Educating Loved Ones:** Help your friends and family understand ARFID so that they can provide more support. Clear communication about your

wants and struggles can increase empathy and create a more supportive workplace.

4. Developing Self-Compassion:

- **Practice Self-care:** Treat yourself with the same care and understanding you would for a friend. Recognize that managing ARFID is difficult, but you are doing your best.
- **Positive Affirmations:** Use positive affirmations to boost self-esteem and decrease self-criticism. Statements like "I am strong and capable," or "I am worthy of love and respect," can help you adjust your perspective.

5. Engaging in Enjoyable Activities:

- **Pursuing Hobbies:** Pursue enjoyable pastimes and hobbies to relax and unwind. This can give a beneficial distraction from food-related anxiety while also improving general happiness.
- **Physical Activity:** Engaging in regular physical activity, such as walking, yoga, or dancing, helps reduce stress and promote mental health. Endorphins are natural mood boosters that are released after exercise.

6. Seeking Professional Help:

- **Therapy:** Working with a therapist, particularly one who specializes in eating disorders, can provide individualized strategies for managing anxiety and emotions. Cognitive-behavioral therapy (CBT) and acceptance and commitment therapy (ACT) are very helpful.
- **Medication:** In rare circumstances, medication may be administered to alleviate anxiety or despair caused by ARFID. Consult a healthcare provider if this choice is necessary.

7. Developing A Structured Routine:

- **Consistent Meal Times:** Setting regular meal and snack times can help to minimize anxiety about eating while also providing a sense of regularity and control.
- **Planning:** To avoid the stress of determining what to eat at the last minute, plan meals and snacks ahead of time. Having a plan might help make mealtimes feel more doable.

8. Practice Gradual Change:

- **Setting Small Goals:** Set small, attainable goals for food and eating. Celebrate your accomplishments, no matter how modest, and utilize each one as a stepping stone to larger changes.
- **Being Patient:** Recognise that progress may be gradual and nonlinear. Be patient with yourself and understand that setbacks are a typical part of the process.

The Importance of Self-Compassion and Acceptance

Living with Avoidant/Restrictive Food Intake Disorder (ARFID) can be stressful and isolating. The route to recovery entails not just modifying eating habits, but also developing a healthy relationship with oneself. Self-compassion and acceptance are essential parts of this process. They provide the emotional support required to handle the challenges of ARFID and enhance general well-being.

Understanding Self-compassion and Acceptance

1. What is self-compassion?

- **Definition:** Self-compassion entails treating oneself with the same love, understanding, and support that one would extend to a good friend. It entails identifying your suffering, admitting your flaws, and responding to yourself with compassion rather than condemnation.

- **Components:** Self-compassion is comprised of three major components: self-kindness, common humanity, and mindfulness. Self-kindness entails being compassionate and understanding towards oneself. Common humanity recognizes that hardship and imperfection are inherent in the human experience. Mindfulness entails remaining present with your feelings without judgment.

2. What is acceptance?

- **Definition:** Acceptance entails acknowledging and embracing all elements of oneself, including your experiences, feelings, and difficulties. It entails letting go of the impulse to modify or control everything and instead seeking tranquility in the current moment.
- **Practice:** Acceptance is about recognizing reality as it is, without resistance. It does not imply giving up on improving your situation, but rather starting from a place of self-awareness and compassion.

The Importance of Self-Compassion and Acceptance in ARFID Recovery

1. Decreased Self-Criticism:

- **Harsh self-judgment:** People with ARFID frequently suffer from self-criticism, feeling ashamed or disappointed by their eating habits. This negative self-talk can worsen anxiety and impede recovery.
- **Kind Self-Talk:** Practicing self-compassion might help you overcome harsh self-judgment. You can alleviate your emotional weight and foster a more helpful inner dialogue by treating yourself with kindness and empathy.

2. Developing Emotional Resilience:

- **Coping with Setbacks:** Recovery from ARFID is a non-linear process with setbacks and hurdles. Self-compassion gives the emotional strength required to get through these ups and downs without feeling overwhelmed or disheartened.
- **Embracing Imperfection:** Acceptance helps you to admit your flaws without letting them define you. It promotes resilience by allowing you to view setbacks as part of the journey rather than failures.

3. Enhancing Self-Worth:

- **Recognizing Your Value:** Self-compassion can help you recognize your intrinsic worth, regardless of your eating choices. It encourages you to see yourself as worthy of love and respect just the way you are.
- **Positive Self-Image:** Acceptance develops a healthy self-image by allowing you to embrace all aspects of yourself, including those with which you may struggle. This holistic self-acceptance can boost your entire sense of worth.

4. Encouraging Healthy Behaviors:

- **Motivating Change:** Self-compassionate persons prioritize their well-being, making them more inclined to engage in healthy behaviors. Rather than pushing change through self-criticism, they are driven by a genuine desire to better their health.
- **Sustainable Recovery:** Acceptance allows you to approach rehabilitation with patience and determination. Accepting where you are in your path allows you to set realistic goals and work towards them at your speed.

Practical Strategies for Developing Self-Compassion and Acceptance.

1. Practicing Mindfulness:

- **Mindful Awareness:** Practice mindfulness through meditation or deep breathing exercises. Mindfulness allows you to be present with your emotions and experiences without judgment, cultivating a caring and welcoming perspective.
- **Body Scan:** Try a body scan meditation to connect with your physical sensations and develop a sense of acceptance for your body.

2. Reframing Self-Talk:

- **Positive Affirmations:** Use positive affirmations to combat negative self-talk. Statements such as "I am worthy of love and respect" or "I am doing my best" will help you adopt a more compassionate attitude towards yourself.
- **Challenge Negative Thoughts:** When you detect self-critical thoughts, question them by asking yourself if you would say the same things to a buddy. Replace these thoughts with more kind and helpful ones.

3. Connecting with Others:

- **Sharing Your Experience:** Share your struggles with trusted friends, family, or support groups. Sharing your stories can make you feel less alone and more understood.
- **Finding Common Humanity:** Realise that you are not alone in your challenges. Many people encounter similar issues, and connecting with others can give you a feeling of shared humanity.

4. Self-Care:

- **Nurturing things:** Find things that bring you joy and relaxation, including reading, wandering in nature, or pursuing a passion. Self-care activities can help you develop a caring relationship with yourself.
- **Physical Self-Care:** Physical self-care, which includes getting enough sleep, eating nutritious foods, and engaging in enjoyable physical activities, promotes general well-being and self-compassion.

5. Seeking Professional Support:

- **Therapy:** Consider engaging with a therapist to build self-acceptance and compassion. Cognitive-behavioral therapy (CBT) and Acceptance and Commitment Therapy (ACT) are two particularly effective therapeutic techniques.
- **Support groups:** Join support groups to connect with others who share your experiences. These gatherings can foster a sense of community and understanding.

Supporting Others Who Have ARFID

Supporting a loved one with Avoidant/Restrictive Food Intake Disorder (ARFID) can be both stressful and gratifying. Your help can have a tremendous impact on their recovery by providing them with the emotional, practical, and moral support they require. Here are some helpful techniques for supporting someone with ARFID.

Educate Yourself About ARFID

1. Understanding The Disorder:

- **Learn about ARFID:** Familiarise yourself with ARFID, its symptoms, and its effects on individuals. Understanding the illness allows you to provide more empathetic and knowledgeable support.

- **Recognize the challenges:** Understand that ARFID is more than just selective eating or a phase; it is a complex eating disorder that necessitates compassion and adequate treatment.

2. Stay informed:

- **Current Research:** Stay up to date on the newest ARFID research and treatment options. This knowledge can help you stay current on effective methods and interventions.
- **Professional Resources:** Use resources from respected organizations like the National Eating Disorders Association (NEDA) and the Academy for Eating Disorders (AED).

Promote Open Communication

1. Encourage Open Dialogue:

- **Create a Safe Space:** Inform your loved one that they may communicate with you about their problems without fear of being judged or criticized. Listen intently and empathetically to their stories and concerns.
- **Be patient:** Recognise that discussing their disorder may be tough. Be patient, and allow them to open up at their speed.

2. Avoid Pressure:

- **Respect Boundaries:** Avoid forcing someone to eat specific meals or modify their eating habits abruptly. Respect their boundaries and collaborate with them to develop gradual, comfortable approaches to addressing their eating difficulties.
- **Validate their feelings:** Recognize and validate their emotions and experiences, even if you don't completely understand them. Statements like "I can see this is very difficult for you" might offer comfort and

support.

Offer practical support

1. Assist with Meals:

- **Meal Planning:** Plan meals that satisfy nutritional needs and accommo-date food preferences and aversions. Work together to strike a balance between introducing new meals and ensuring safety.
- **Cooking Together:** If it is comfortable for them, prepare meals together. This can reduce tension and make eating more enjoyable.

2. Foster a Supportive Environment:

- **Avoid Negative Comments:** Refrain from making negative comments about food, eating habits, or body image. Create a happy and encouraging workplace that values progress and effort above perfection.
- **Encourage positive experiences:** Encourage them to participate in social activities and events that are not centered on food. Encourage hobbies and activities that they enjoy that can help them feel less anxious.

Encourage professional help

1. Advocate for Treatment:

- **Suggest Professional Support:** Encourage seeking professional care for ARFID, including therapists, nutritionists, and doctors. If they are comfortable, offer to assist them in finding resources or to accompany them to appointments.
- **Respect their decisions:** While advocating for professional aid is crucial, remember to respect their autonomy and treatment decisions. Assist them

in identifying the appropriate professionals and therapy techniques for their requirements.

2. Collaborate with professionals:

- **Coordinate Care:** Collaborate with their treatment team to ensure consistent support. This could include attending family therapy sessions or following the advice of their healthcare specialists.
- **Follow Through:** Encourage them to follow through on treatment plans and interventions. Provide encouragement and responsibility without being overwhelming.

Be aware of your well-being

1. Set boundaries:

- **Know Your Limitations:** Supporting someone with ARFID can be emotionally draining. Set appropriate limits to ensure that you are caring for your well-being.
- **Seek Help:** Consider attending a support group for family and friends of people who have eating problems. Connecting with individuals in similar situations might provide useful information and emotional support.

2. Practice self-care:

- **Take time for yourself:** Engage in activities that you enjoy and will help you relax. Taking care of your own mental and emotional health is essential for being a good carer for your loved one.
- **Seek Professional Help:** If you're struggling to cope with the emotional demands of caring for someone with ARFID, go to a therapist or counselor.

III

Part 3: Tools and Techniques for Overcoming ARFID

5

Chapter 5: The Role of Healthcare Professionals in ARFID Recovery

Therapists, Nutritionists, and Doctors

herapists play an important role in the treatment of Avoidant/Restrictive Food Intake Disorder. They provide psychological support and techniques to address the underlying causes of the illness and assist clients in developing healthier eating habits. Cognitive Behavioural Therapy (CBT) and Exposure Therapy are two common therapeutic modalities utilized in ARFID treatment.

Cognitive behaviour therapy (CBT)

1. Understanding the CBT:

- **Definition:** Cognitive Behavioural Therapy is a planned, time-limited psychotherapy that seeks to change patterns of thinking or behavior that are causing people's issues, thereby altering how they feel.
- **Goals:** The primary goals of CBT in ARFID treatment are to identify and

challenge negative thought patterns about food, eating, and body image, and to replace them with more positive and realistic ones.

2. CBT Techniques for ARFID Treatment:

- **Cognitive Restructuring:** Cognitive restructuring entails identifying and confronting illogical or damaging attitudes towards food and eating. For example, someone with ARFID may assume that trying new foods is unsafe. A therapist can help individuals reframe this thinking by reviewing data and forming a more balanced viewpoint.
- **Behavioral Strategies:** These include setting progressive, attainable goals for experimenting with new meals and developing eating confidence. Therapists may employ tactics like reward systems to reinforce positive eating habits.
- **Skill Building:** Therapists offer coping methods for controlling food-related anxiety and stress. This could include relaxation techniques, awareness, and problem-solving abilities to deal with situations that cause ARFID symptoms.
- **Monitoring and Reflection:** Clients may be requested to keep a food diary to record their eating habits and thoughts about food. This helps to identify triggers and track improvements over time.

Exposure Therapy

1. Understanding Exposure Therapy:

- **Definition:** Exposure Therapy is a behavioral treatment that progressively and methodically exposes individuals to feared things or events, such as specific meals or eating contexts, to lessen anxiety and avoidance behaviors.
- **Goal:** To minimize fear and anxiety associated with specific meals or eating situations, and progressively increase exposure in a regulated and

supportive manner.

2. Exposure Therapy Techniques for ARFID Treatment:

- **Hierarchy of Exposure:** Therapists and clients collaborate to establish a hierarchy of feared meals or eating scenarios, beginning with the least anxiety-inducing and advancing to the most stressful.
- **Gradual Exposure:** Beginning with less dreaded foods or situations, people are gradually exposed to these triggers in a controlled manner. For example, they may begin by being in the same room as the meal, then advance to touching it and finally eating it.
- **Performed Practice:** Exposure is performed several times to help lessen fear and increase confidence. Repeated exposure teaches the brain that the feared food or situation is not as hazardous as it first appears.
- **Coping Mechanisms:** During exposure, therapists assist clients in managing anxiety with coping mechanisms such as deep breathing, mindfulness, and positive visualization.
- **Support and Encouragement:** Therapists provide continuous support and encouragement, assisting clients in reflecting on their progress and reinforcing their efforts.

The Combined Approach

1. Integrating CBT with Exposure Therapy:

- **Comprehensive Treatment Plan:** Combining CBT and Exposure Therapy allows for a more thorough treatment plan. While CBT tackles the underlying cognitive and emotional elements of ARFID, Exposure Therapy aims to reduce the behavioral avoidance of specific foods.
- **Holistic Support:** This integrated approach addresses both the ideas and behaviors that contribute to ARFID, resulting in a more comprehensive and effective therapy.

The therapist-client relationship

1. Building Trust:

- **Therapeutic Alliance:** A strong, trustworthy relationship between therapist and client is essential. Therapists establish a safe, nonjudgmental environment in which clients can communicate their anxieties and challenges.
- **Empathy and Understanding:** Therapists demonstrate empathy and understanding by validating their clients' experiences and feelings. This support is critical for making customers feel listened to and supported.

2. Individualised Treatment:

- **Tailored Approach:** Therapists adjust their approach to match the unique needs and circumstances of each client with ARFID. This could imply focusing on cognitive strategies for some individuals and exposure techniques for others.
- **Flexible Goals:** Therapists collaborate with clients to establish flexible and realistic goals, adjusting the treatment plan as needed based on the client's progress and feedback.

The Role of a Registered Dietitian in Creating a Personalized Meal Plan

Registered dietitians (RDs) play an important role in the treatment and management of avoidant/restrictive food intake disorder (ARFID). They contribute a specialized understanding of nutrition and dietetics, which is critical for addressing the specific dietary issues that people with ARFID confront. Their responsibilities go beyond simple meal preparation; they also provide specialized nutritional advice, education, and assistance to help people achieve a balanced diet and enhance their overall health.

Understanding the role of a registered dietitian

1. Knowledge of Nutrition:

- **Specialized Training:** RDs have considerable nutrition education and training, allowing them to grasp the intricacies of dietary demands and how numerous circumstances, including medical illnesses such as ARFID, affect nutrition.
- **Evidence-Based Practice:** They use evidence-based techniques to deliver the best effective nutritional therapies and support.

2. Holistic Approach:

- **Comprehensive Assessment:** RDs undertake extensive examinations of an individual's dietary habits, nutritional status, and health history to better understand their needs.
- **Collaborative Care:** They frequently work as part of a multidisciplinary team, partnering with therapists, doctors, and other healthcare professionals to deliver comprehensive care.

Developing a Personalized Meal Plan

1. Initial Assessment:

- **Nutritional Evaluation:** The RD assesses the individual's current consumption to discover deficits or imbalances. This could include checking food diaries, conducting interviews, and sometimes running biochemical tests.
- **Understanding preferences and aversions:** The registered dietitian identifies unique dietary preferences, sensory aversions, and eating-related concerns. This information is critical for creating a meal plan

that the person can stick to.

2. Setting Nutritional Goals:

- **Individualized Goals:** RDs establish personalized and realistic nutritional objectives based on evaluation results. These objectives are intended to alleviate deficiencies, promote balanced nutrition, and meet the individual's unique demands and problems.
- **Short-Term and Long-Term Planning:** The RD establishes both short-term and long-term objectives, ensuring that the meal plan evolves as the individual progresses.

3. Creating the Meal Plan:

- **Balanced Nutrition:** The RD creates a balanced meal plan that includes macronutrients (carbohydrates, proteins, fats) and micronutrients (vitamins and minerals) for optimal health.
- **Incorporating Safe Meals:** The meal plan contains safe meals that the individual is comfortable eating while progressively introducing new foods to broaden their nutritional range.
- **Adaptation to Preferences:** The RD tailors the meal plan to the individual's taste preferences, increasing the likelihood that they will adhere to it. For example, if the individual prefers bland textures, the RD will include more foods with those textures at first.

4. Addressing Nutritional Deficiencies:

- **Supplementation:** If a person has serious nutritional deficiencies that cannot be fulfilled by food alone, a registered dietitian may recommend appropriate supplements.
- **Education:** The RD teaches the individual about the importance of specific nutrients and how to include them in their diet, resulting in a better understanding and appreciation for balanced nutrition.

Providing Ongoing Support and Education

1. Regular Monitoring and Adjustment:

- **Continuous Evaluation:** The RD periodically monitors the individual's progress, adjusting the meal plan as needed to ensure it remains effective and meets their changing needs.
- **Feedback and Encouragement:** Regular follow-up sessions allow for feedback, address any issues or concerns that the individual may have, and offer encouragement and inspiration.

2. Education and Empowerment:

- **Nutritional Knowledge:** The RD educates individuals on nutrition and healthy eating habits, enabling them to make informed diet decisions.
- **Cooking Skills:** They may provide practical advice and recommendations on food preparation and cooking procedures, increasing the individual's confidence in the kitchen.

3. Supportive Environment:

- **Positive Reinforcement:** The RD promotes progress and little success, building a positive relationship with food.
- **Coping tactics:** They offer tactics for dealing with food-related anxiety and obstacles, such as mindful eating or relaxation exercises before meals.

Cooperating with the Treatment Team

1. Integrated Care:

- **Working with Therapists:** RDs work closely with therapists to ensure the dietary plan complements psychological treatment, including adding exposure therapy approaches into meal planning.

- **Medical Oversight:** They work with doctors to monitor the individual's physical health and ensure that any medical difficulties associated with ARFID are treated immediately.

2. Family Involvement:

- **Education for Caregivers:** The RD educates and supports carers to better understand their loved one's nutritional needs and provide effective support.
- **Family Meals:** They may provide advice on how to prepare family meals that satisfy the individual's dietary needs while being pleasurable for everyone.

The Role of a Doctor in Monitoring Physical Health and Addressing Medical Concerns

Doctors play an important role in the treatment of Avoidant/Restrictive Food Intake illness (ARFID), providing necessary medical oversight to guarantee the physical health and well-being of those suffering from this illness. Their tasks include ARFID diagnosis, physical health monitoring, medical problem resolution, and care coordination with other healthcare experts.

Diagnosing ARFID

1. Comprehensive evaluation:

- **Initial Assessment:** Doctors undertake rigorous evaluations to diagnose ARFID. This includes obtaining a thorough medical history, analyzing eating habits, and recognizing any physical symptoms associated with the disorder.

- **Differential Diagnosis:** They distinguish ARFID from other medical diseases or eating disorders that exhibit similar symptoms, such as anorexia nervosa or gastrointestinal disorders.

2. Diagnostic criteria:

- **Using recognized Criteria:** To diagnose ARFID, doctors apply recognized diagnostic criteria from the Diagnostic and Statistical Manual of Mental Disorders (DSM-5). This includes evaluating concerns such as severe weight loss, dietary deficiencies, reliance on nutritional supplements, and problems with psychosocial functioning.

Monitoring Physical Health

1.Regular Check-Ups:

- **Routine Examinations:** Regular medical check-ups are essential for people with ARFID to maintain their overall health and spot potential issues early.
- **Tracking Growth and Development:** To ensure that children and adolescents are on track, doctors regularly monitor growth and development characteristics such as height, weight, and body mass index (BMI).

2. Nutritional Status:

- **Assessing Nutrient Levels:** Doctors assess nutrient levels using blood testing to detect deficits in vitamins, minerals, and vital substances.
- **Hydration and Electrolyte Balance:** They monitor hydration and electrolyte balance, which are critical for overall health and avoiding issues.

Addressing Medical Concerns

1. Treating Malnutrition:

- **Nutritional Interventions:** Doctors may recommend nutritional supplements or medical nutrition therapy to address vitamin deficits. This may include high-calorie supplements, multivitamins, or particular nutrients such as iron or calcium.
- **Hospitalization:** In severe cases where malnutrition offers an immediate health danger, hospitalization may be required for intense nutritional care and monitoring.

2. Managing Physical Symptoms:

- **Gastrointestinal Issues:** ARFID patients frequently have gastrointestinal issues including constipation, abdominal discomfort, and bloating. To control these symptoms, doctors prescribe suitable therapies, such as drugs or dietary adjustments.
- **Other Medical diseases:** They also treat any co-occurring medical diseases caused by poor nutrition, such as infections, hormonal imbalances, or bone health difficulties.

3. Avoiding Long-term Complications:

- **Bone Health:** Doctors monitor bone density, particularly in children and adolescents, to avoid long-term issues including osteoporosis and fractures. They may suggest calcium and vitamin D supplements if necessary.
- **Immune Function:** They ensure that the individual's immune system is functioning properly, as malnutrition can impair immunity and make them more susceptible to illnesses.

Coordinating Care

1. Multidisciplinary Team:

- **Collaborative Approach:** Doctors collaborate with therapists, dietitians, and other professionals to provide complete therapy to persons with ARFID.
- **Integrated Treatment Plans:** They help to create and implement integrated treatment plans that address both the physical and psychological elements of ARFID.

2. Family Involvement:

- **Educating Families:** Doctors educate families on the medical aspects of ARFID, emphasizing the necessity of following treatment plans and identifying indicators of problems.
- **Support and Guidance:** They help families negotiate the obstacles of managing ARFID and ensure their loved one's well-being.

Providing ongoing support

1. Monitoring Progress:

- **Follow-up Appointments:** Regular follow-up appointments enable doctors to track the patient's progress, change therapies as appropriate, and address any new or persistent medical concerns.
- **Encouragement and Motivation:** Doctors can help persons with ARFID stay on track with their treatment and make good adjustments in their eating habits.

2. Crisis Management:

- **Addressing Acute Issues:** In the event of an ARFID-related medical emergency, clinicians provide rapid care to stabilize the patient's health.
- **Coordinating Emergency Care:** They work with emergency services and specialists to provide complete care during a crisis.

Developing a Personalized Treatment Plan

Treating Avoidant/Restrictive Food Intake Disorder (ARFID) necessitates a multidisciplinary strategy that includes medical, nutritional, and psychological treatments. This comprehensive approach is required to address the disorder's complex and diverse character.

Medical interventions

1. Nutritional Support:

- **Supplementation:** Doctors may provide nutritional supplements to correct deficits. These can comprise vitamins, minerals, or high-calorie supplements to ensure that the individual gets enough nutrients.
- **Medical Nutrition Therapy:** In severe circumstances, enteral nutrition (tube feeding) may be required to maintain the individual's nutritional condition.

2. Monitoring and Management:

- **Regular Check-Ups:** Regular medical exams track an individual's physical health, growth, and development.
- **Managing Complications:** Medical practitioners address any complications caused by malnutrition, such as gastrointestinal problems or decreased immunity.

Nutritional Interventions

1. Personalised Meal Plans:

- **Registered Dietitian:** A registered dietitian creates meal plans based on the needs and interests of individuals with ARFID. This includes incorporating safe foods while progressively introducing new ones.
- **Nutritional Education:** Dietitians teach people and families the value of balanced nutrition and a diverse diet.

2.Addressing Sensory Issues:

- **Sensory Integration Therapy:** Dietitians and occupational therapists use desensitization strategies to assist clients become more comfortable with various food textures, odors, and tastes.
- **Gradual Exposure:** To lessen sensory aversions, introduce new meals gradually and in a controlled manner. Additionally, psychological interventions might be used.

Psychological Interventions

1. Cognitive Behavioural Therapy (CBT):

- **CBT Techniques:** CBT techniques help individuals identify and change negative thoughts about food and eating. It can help with anxiety, fear of choking, and other psychological issues that contribute to ARFID.
- **Exposure Therapy:** This method entails gradually exposing people to feared foods in a safe and supportive atmosphere to diminish anxiety and avoidance behaviors.

2. Family-based therapy (FBT):

- **Involving Family:** FBT involves family members in the treatment process by teaching them about ARFID and enabling them to help their loved one's recovery.
- **Meal Support:** Families are educated to assist with meals, allowing the individual with ARFID to eat in a more structured and supportive setting.

3. Dialectical Behaviour Therapy (DBT):

- **Emotional Regulation:** DBT strategies assist patients in managing intense emotions that may interfere with eating, such as anxiety or discomfort.
- **Mindfulness Practices:** Mindfulness techniques are used to promote present-moment awareness and minimize eating-related stress.

Behavioral Interventions

1. Positive Reinforcement:

- **Reward Systems:** Reward systems can motivate people to try new meals and adopt healthier eating habits. Rewards might be non-food in nature, such as more playtime or a favorite hobby.
- **Behavioral Contracts:** Using behavioral contracts to provide clear goals and rewards can help motivate and structure the treatment process.

2. Exposure and Response Prevention (ERP):

- **Gradual Exposure:** Gradual exposure to feared foods reduces anxiety and increases food acceptance.
- **Supportive Environment:** This procedure is frequently carried out in a supportive and regulated environment to ensure safety and comfort.

Integrative and holistic approaches

1. Mindfulness and Relaxation:

- **Mindfulness Techniques:** Practices like mindful eating can reduce anxiety and improve one's connection with food.
- **Relaxation Exercises:** Deep breathing, progressive muscle relaxation, and guided imagery can all help to reduce eating-related stress and anxiety.

2. Occupational Therapy:

- **Skill Development:** Occupational therapists help individuals improve their abilities in food preparation, meal planning, and eating in various settings.
- **Sensory Integration:** They also treat sensory processing disorders that might lead to food avoidance and aversions.

Collaborative and Multidisciplinary Care

1. Team Approach:

- **Integrated Care:** To effectively treat ARFID, healthcare experts such as doctors, dietitians, therapists, and occupational therapists collaborate to provide complete therapy.
- **Regular Communication:** Team members must communicate consistently to ensure that the treatment plan is cohesive and that all areas of the individual's health and well-being are addressed.

2. Ongoing Support:

- **Follow-Up Care:** Regular follow-up consultations with healthcare providers are essential for monitoring progress and making adjustments to the treatment plan.

- **Support Groups:** Joining a support group can provide individuals and families with further encouragement, understanding, and shared experiences.

Developing a Treatment Plan Based on Your Individual Presentation

Developing a successful treatment plan for Avoidant/Restrictive Food Intake Disorder (ARFID) necessitates a tailored strategy that takes into account each individual's specific requirements, problems, and aspirations. Here's how to create a personalised treatment plan that addresses the unique elements of your ARFID presentation.

Initial Assessment

1. Comprehensive Evaluation:

- **Medical History:** A detailed medical history is sought to determine any underlying health concerns, dietary deficits, and past attempts to manage eating disorders.
- **Psychological Assessment:** An assessment of psychological issues such as anxiety, depression, and any co-occurring mental health conditions aids in the identification of the emotional elements of ARFID.
- **Nutritional Assessment:** A dietitian evaluates current eating patterns, dietary preferences, and nutritional intake to identify shortfalls and areas for improvement.

2. Identifying key issues:

- **Presenting symptoms:** Determine the primary symptoms of ARFID, which may include sensory aversions, fear of choking, or a lack of interest in food.

- **Impact on daily life:** Evaluate the impact of ARFID on daily functioning, such as social interactions, academic or work performance, and general quality of life.

Setting Goals

1. Short-term Goals:

- **Immediate Health Concerns:** Address immediate health concerns, such as maintaining weight, fixing nutrient deficits, and controlling physical symptoms such as gastrointestinal distress.
- **Building Trust:** Create a therapeutic connection based on trust and understanding, so that the individual feels supported and motivated to participate in therapy.

2. Long-term goal:

- **Nutritional Rehabilitation:** To improve emotional well-being, aim for balanced and diverse nutrition, including widening the spectrum of acceptable meals. Additionally, address any underlying psychological concerns that may be causing anxiety about eating.
- **Improving Quality of Life:** Set goals for social participation, healthy eating habits, and general life satisfaction.

Adjusting the Approach

1. Sensory Sensitivities:

- **Desensitization Techniques:** Gradual exposure to various food textures, scents, and flavors can help lessen sensory aversions. This can be accomplished through systematic desensitization, in which the individual is gradually exposed to novel sensory stimuli in a controlled environment.

- **Safe Food Expansion:** Begin with safe foods and progressively add similar items to extend the diet without overwhelming the individual.

2. Fear of Choking:

- **Safe Eating Practices:** To address choking fears, teach safe eating techniques including taking tiny pieces, chewing properly, and using supportive seating and utensils.
- **CBT for Anxiety:** Use cognitive behavioral therapy (CBT) to alleviate the anxiety associated with choking, assisting the individual in developing healthy thought patterns and coping methods.

3. Lack of Interest in Food:

- **Stimulating Appetite:** To promote appetite, try scheduling frequent meals, providing a pleasant dining environment, and using appetite-enhancing vitamins as needed.
- **Exploring Food Variety:** Encourage the exploration of new foods in a relaxed setting, concentrating on the sensory and social enjoyment of eating rather than just nutrition.

Interventions and Therapies

1. Medical and Nutritional Support:

- **Regular Monitoring:** Schedule regular check-ups to monitor physical health, nutritional status, and growth (in children and adolescents).
- **Customized Meal Plans:** Work with a registered dietitian to create meal plans that meet nutritional needs while considering food preferences and aversions.

2. Psychological Therapies:

- **CBT and Exposure Therapy:** CBT and Exposure Therapy can help challenge and transform negative ideas about food and eating. Exposure treatment helps to lessen fear and avoidance behaviours.
- **Family-Based Therapy (FBT):** Involves family members in the therapy process to offer support, understanding, and encouragement.

3. Behavioural Strategy:

- **Positive Reinforcement:** Use positive reinforcement to encourage people to try new foods and adopt healthy eating habits. Rewards should be non-food based and meaningful to the individual.
- **Behavioral Contracts:** Create behavioral contracts that outline precise goals and rewards, motivating and guiding progress.

Building a Support System

1. Involving Family and Friends:

- **Education and Training:** Educate and train them on ARFID to help them comprehend the issues and provide necessary support.
- **Supportive Environment:** Create a welcoming and nonjudgmental eating environment at home and in social situations.

2. Professional Collaboration:

- **Multidisciplinary Team:** Collaborate with a multidisciplinary team of healthcare experts, including doctors, dietitians, therapists, and occupational therapists, to deliver comprehensive care.
- **Regular Communication:** Maintain regular communication with all members of the treatment team to establish a cohesive and coordinated

strategy.

Monitoring and Adjusting the Plan

1. Regular Review:

- **Progress Evaluation:** Evaluate progress towards goals and alter treatment plans based on individual responses.
- **Feedback Loop:** Encourage the individual and their family to provide feedback so that improvements may be made and the treatment remains effective and helpful.

2. Flexibility and Patience:

- **Adapting Strategies:** Adapt techniques based on changing demands and conditions.
- **Patience and Persistence:** Recognise that improvement may be delayed and non-linear, necessitating patience and perseverance from both the individual and the treatment team.

The Importance of Collaboration Between Patient, Therapist, and Family

Collaboration between the patient, therapist, and family is essential for the successful treatment of Avoidant/Restrictive Food Intake Disorder (ARFID). This integrated approach guarantees that all parts of the condition are treated, offering comprehensive care to the patient. Here's why collaboration is important and how it may be efficiently applied.

Comprehensive Understanding of ARFID

1. Comprehensive Perspective:

- **Patient Insight:** The patient offers firsthand information about their ARFID-related experiences, obstacles, and sentiments, which is critical for developing a personalized treatment plan.
- **Therapist Expertise:** Therapists contribute professional knowledge, evidence-based solutions, and therapy procedures to treat the psychological components of ARFID.
- **Family Support:** Family members provide emotional and practical support, establishing a loving environment that promotes healing.

2. Coordinated Care:

- **Shared Information:** Regular communication among patients, therapists, and families promotes a unified approach to therapy.
- **Unified Goals:** Setting common goals and expectations helps to align efforts and develops a sense of community and mutual support.

Enhanced Treatment Results

1. Emotional and Practical Support:

- **Emotional Stability:** Having a supportive family can provide emotional stability and encouragement, which is important for the patient's mental health and motivation.
- **Practical Help:** Family members can help with food preparation, providing a positive eating environment, and managing daily routines, making the practical aspects of treatment easier to manage.

2. Improved Treatment Adherence:

- **Accountability:** Regular involvement of family and therapist promotes patient accountability and adherence to treatment plans and activities.
- **Consistent Support:** Continuous support from both the therapist and the family lowers feelings of isolation and increases the possibility of long-term engagement in the recovery process.

Addressing Emotional and Behavioural Challenges

1. Managing Anxiety and Emotions:

- **Therapeutic Interventions:** Therapists employ cognitive behavioral therapy (CBT) to address anxiety, dread of eating, and other emotional issues related to ARFID.
- **Family Understanding:** Teaching family members about ARFID and its emotional effects allows them to respond with empathy and provide appropriate emotional support.

2. Behavioural Modification:

- **Reinforcement Strategies:** To promote healthier eating habits and lessen avoidance, therapists and family members can work together to apply positive reinforcement tactics.
- **Consistent Environment:** A consistent approach to therapy sessions and the home environment supports new behaviors and coping strategies, facilitating long-term transformation.

Creating a supportive environment

1. Creating a Positive Eating Experience:

- **Safe Spaces:** Families can create secure, non-judgmental eating environments to alleviate stress and anxiety during meals.
- **Encouraging Exploration:** Therapists advise families on how to help patients sample new foods and increase their dietary repertoire in a progressive, non-threatening manner.

2. Education and Empowerment:

- **Family Education:** Giving families knowledge about ARFID, its causes, and treatment options enables them to be effective supporters in the recovery process.
- **Patient Empowerment:** Involving the patient in decision-making and goal-setting gives them a sense of agency and empowerment, which increases their motivation to heal.

Flexibility and Adaptation

1. Responsive adjustments:

- **Feedback Loop:** Continuous feedback from the patient, therapist, and family enables rapid revisions to the treatment plan, ensuring that it remains relevant and effective.
- **Adapting Strategies:** The ability to adapt therapeutic approaches and support strategies to the changing demands of the patient improves the treatment's overall effectiveness.

2. Long-term Support:

- **Sustainable Engagement:** Ongoing collaboration ensures that the patient receives ongoing support even after the initial treatment goals are fulfilled, thereby reducing relapse and promoting long-term well-being.
- **Life Transitions:** As the patient moves through different life stages, the collaborative approach allows the support system to adapt to new problems and demands.

Building a Support System: The Importance of Family and Friends

Understanding Avoidant/Restrictive Food Intake Disorder (ARFID) can be difficult for family and friends, but their help is essential for successful treatment and recovery. Educating others who are close to someone with ARFID promotes a supportive environment and creates empathy, understanding, and effective help. Here's how to teach your relatives and friends about ARFID.

Basics of ARFID

1. Defining ARFID:

- **What is ARFID?** Explain that ARFID is an eating disorder characterized by the avoidance of particular foods or a lack of interest in eating, which results in major nutritional deficits and has an impact on physical health.
- **Common misconceptions:** Clarify that ARFID is more than just picky eating; it is a significant mental health disorder that requires expert help.

2. Symptoms and behavior:

- **Varied Presentations:** ARFID can show in a variety of ways, including sensory aversions (a distaste for specific textures, scents, or tastes), fear of choking, and a general lack of interest in food.
- **Impact on Daily Life:** Explain how ARFID affects daily activities, social

relationships, and general quality of life, including any potential physical or emotional health consequences.

Emotional and Psychological Impact

1. Understanding Emotional Struggles:

- **worry and Fear:** People with ARFID often experience intense worry and fear associated with eating, which can be debilitating.
- **Emotional Toll:** Discuss how ARFID can cause emotions of shame, guilt, loneliness, and despair, affecting self-esteem and mental health.

2. Empathy and Support:

- **Non-judgmental attitude:** Encourage family and friends to be nonjudgmental and sensitive, recognizing that ARFID is not a choice, but rather a condition that requires compassion and support.
- **Active Listening:** Emphasise the significance of active listening, which allows people with ARFID to share their emotions and challenges without fear of being judged or dismissed.

Practical Ways to Support

1. Creating a Supportive Environment:

- **Positive Meal Times:** Maintain a calm, positive, and pressure-free environment during meals. Avoid making forceful or critical comments about food.
- **Flexibility and Patience:** Encourage patience and flexibility in meal planning by accommodating the individual's safe meals while gradually introducing new foods without pressure.

2. Involvement in Treatment:

- **Collaborative Approach:** Explain the advantages of a collaborative approach that includes patients, families, and healthcare professionals. Emphasize the importance of family support in therapy.
- **Education on Treatment Tactics:** Inform family members about treatment tactics such as cognitive behavioral therapy (CBT), exposure therapy, and dietary counselling so that they may comprehend the therapeutic process.

Resources and Further Learning

1. Informational Materials:

- **Books and Articles:** Recommend books, articles, and online resources for comprehensive information about ARFID, including symptoms, treatment choices, and support strategies.
- **Educational Workshops:** Attend workshops or webinars offered by professionals who specialize in ARFID and eating disorders to acquire better knowledge and practical advice.

2. Professional Guidance:

- **Therapist Involvement:** Involve family and friends in therapy sessions and seek guidance from therapists on how to support the individual with ARFID.
- **Support Groups:** Join support groups for relatives of people with eating disorders, which provide a forum for sharing experiences, gaining insights, and receiving emotional support.

Encourage open communication.

1. Building Trust:

- **Open Dialogue:** Encourage open and honest communication regarding ARFID, ensuring individuals feel secure to share their experiences, problems, and progress without fear of judgment.
- **Check-Ins:** Make regular contact with the individual to discuss their feelings and needs, ensuring they feel heard and supported throughout their recovery journey.

2. Addressing Concerns:

- **Healthy Boundaries:** Discuss the significance of maintaining healthy boundaries, respecting the individual's autonomy, and balancing support with independence.
- **Problem-Solving Together:** Work together to solve any obstacles or setbacks productively and collaboratively, instilling a spirit of collaboration and mutual support.

Enlisting Their Support During Treatment

Enlisting the help of family and friends throughout therapy for Avoidant/Restrictive Food Intake Disorder (ARFID) can greatly speed up the recovery process. Their engagement offers emotional support, practical aid, and reinforcement of therapy procedures. Here's how to effectively enlist and use the support of loved ones while in therapy.

Understanding the Role of Support

1. Emotional Anchors:

- **Emotional Stability:** Family and friends can offer emotional support and understanding during difficult times.
- **Positive Reinforcement:** Their support and positive reinforcement can help the patient gain confidence and motivation to participate in treatment.

2. Practical Assistance:

- **Meal Preparation:** Family members can assist with meal planning and preparation, ensuring the patient has access to safe and healthy meals.
- **Routine Management:** Helping patients manage their everyday routines and duties can minimize stress and allow them to focus on their rehabilitation.

Educating your loved ones

1. Providing Information:

- **Understanding ARFID:** Ensure family and friends understand ARFID, including symptoms, causes, and treatment options.
- **Educational Resources:** Share books, articles, and credible online resources to help them expand their knowledge and comprehension.

2. Setting Expectations:

- **Realistic Goals:** Establish reasonable goals and recognize that healing from ARFID is a gradual process.

- **Role Clarity:** Clarify the duties and responsibilities of family and friends in the treatment process, so that everyone understands how to best help the patient.

Creating a supportive environment

1. Positive Meal Times:

- **Calm Atmosphere:** Create a peaceful and cheerful atmosphere during meals, eliminating pressure, criticism, or bad remarks regarding eating habits.
- **Safe Foods:** Respect and accommodate the patient's safe foods while progressively introducing new ones according to the treatment plan.

2. Emotional Support:

- **Active Listening:** Teach the value of active listening, which allows patients to communicate their thoughts and challenges without interruption or judgment.
- **Empathy and Patience:** Encourage empathy and patience while realizing that ARFID-related behaviors are not choices, but rather symptoms of the condition.

Practical Strategies for Support

1. Participation in Therapy:

- **Family Sessions:** Involve family members in treatment sessions to receive direct instruction from the therapist and address family issues that may affect the patient's rehabilitation.
- **Communication with Professionals:** Keep open lines of communication

with the patient's healthcare team to ensure that family members are informed and on board with the treatment plan.

2. Daily Encouragement:

- **Celebrating Progress:** Celebrate modest triumphs and milestones in inpatient rehabilitation to reinforce positive behaviors and development.
- **Consistent Support:** Offer consistent support while acknowledging that there may be setbacks and problems along the path and that perseverance and patience are essential.

Building a Positive and Encouraging Environment

Creating a good and encouraging environment is critical for helping someone with Avoidant/Restrictive Food Intake Disorder (ARFID). This loving environment can considerably aid in their recovery by supporting emotional well-being and encouraging healthy eating habits. Here are some ideas for creating such an environment at home and within the larger support network.

cultivating a positive atmosphere

1. Encouragement vs Criticism:

- **Positive reinforcement:** Instead of criticizing losses, celebrate minor triumphs and beneficial behaviors. Praise the person for trying new foods or making progress in therapy.
- **Avoid Negative Comments:** Avoid making nasty or judgmental comments about their eating habits or food choices. This reduces anxiety and promotes a sense of safety and acceptance.

2. Empathy and understanding:

- **Active Listening:** Active listening entails paying full attention to the speaker, respecting their feelings, and validating their experiences without passing judgment.
- **Express Empathy:** Empathy is demonstrated by exhibiting sympathy and compassion for the issues they experience. Statements like, "I understand how difficult this is for you, and I'm here to support you," can be incredibly reassuring.

Creating A Safe Eating Environment

1. Safe and Calm Mealtimes:

- **Relaxed Setting:** Set a peaceful and relaxed tone throughout meals. Avoid distractions like TV or angry talks, which can exacerbate tension and anxiety.
- **Schedule and Consistency:** Create a consistent meal schedule to provide predictability and stability, which can help minimize anxiety associated with eating.

2. Respecting Food Preferences

- **Safe Foods:** Incorporate the individual's safe foods into meals and respect their tastes while progressively introducing new foods as prescribed in the treatment plan.
- **Gentle Introduction:** Introduce new meals in a non-threatening, pressure-free manner. Use positive reinforcement and combine new and safe meals to make the process less scary.

Encouraging Positive Interactions

1. Supportive Communication:

- **Positive Language:** Use pleasant and encouraging words while talking about food and eating. Avoid phrases that may indicate judgment or pressure.
- **Open Dialogue:** Maintain an open discourse in which individuals feel free to communicate their views and feelings regarding food and their eating experiences.

2. Engaging Activities:

- **Involvement in Meal Prep:** Involve individuals in meal planning and preparation to enhance their comfort and familiarity with food. This can also give a sensation of control and accomplishment.
- **Family Meals:** Encourage family meals, in which everyone eats together in a friendly and cheerful environment. This can help to normalize the eating experience and create a sense of belonging.

Developing Resilience and Coping Skills

1. Developing Coping Mechanisms:

- **Stress Management:** To help manage food-related anxiety, teach and encourage stress management practices such as mindfulness, deep breathing exercises, and other relaxation approaches.
- **Therapeutic Support:** Encourage involvement in treatment to create coping techniques for dealing with the emotional components of ARFID. Encourage their attendance and interest in therapy sessions.

2. Promoting Self-Compassion:

- **Self-Acceptance:** Remind them that progress is an ongoing process and that setbacks are normal.
- **Positive Self-Talk:** Encourage them to use positive self-talk, emphasizing on their strengths and accomplishments rather than their challenges.

Supporting Long-Term Recovery

1. Consistent Support:

- **Ongoing Encouragement:** Offer continued encouragement and support, even after initial treatment goals are achieved. Continuous support helps to sustain development and avoid relapse.
- **Regular Check-Ins:** Check in with the individual regularly to learn about their sentiments, progress, and any obstacles they may be encountering, demonstrating that you are there for them long term.

2. Professional guidance:

- **Collaborative Care:** Collaborate with healthcare providers to ensure that the patient receives thorough care. This involves regular visits with their therapist, dietician, and doctor.
- **Education Resources:** Learn more about ARFID and its treatment by using educational resources. This allows you to better support and understand the individual's requirements.

6

Chapter 6: Practical Strategies for Managing ARFID Symptoms

Desensitization Techniques for Overcoming Aversions

Understanding the sensory stimuli linked with food is critical for treating Avoidant/Restrictive Food Intake Disorder (ARFID). Sensory sensitivities might impair an individual's ability to consume a diverse and balanced diet. Identifying these triggers will help you develop strategies for managing and eventually reducing their influence. This is a complete guide on detecting and treating sensory triggers relating to texture, smell, and appearance.

Understanding Sensory Triggers

1. The Function of Sensory Sensitivities:

- **Definition:** Sensory triggers in ARFID are specific qualities of food that elicit discomfort or aversion, such as texture, smell, or look.
- **Impact on Eating:** These triggers might cause people to avoid particular

meals, limit their dietary variety, and develop nutritional deficiencies.

Identifying Texture Triggers

1. Common Texture Sensitivities:

- **Crunchy or Hard Foods:** Crunchy or firm meals might be difficult to chew for certain people, so they avoid them.
- **Slimy or Soft Foods:** Some people dislike slimy or overly soft textures, including some fruits or cooked vegetables.

2. Observations and Documentation:

- **Food journal:** Keep a detailed food journal to track which textures are bothersome. Take note of any physical symptoms (gagging, spitting out food) and mental responses (worry, dissatisfaction).
- **Sensory Testing:** Sensory testing involves introducing a variety of meals with varying textures in a controlled environment to examine reactions. This aids in determining specific textures that cause discomfort.

3. Engage the Individual:

- **Direct Communication:** Ask the person about their preferences and aversions. Ask explicit inquiries about how various materials make them feel.
- **Comfortable Environment:** Make sure the talk takes place in a pleasant and friendly environment to encourage openness and honesty.

Identifying Smell Trigger

1. Common Smell Sensibilities:

- **Strong Odours:** Foods with strong odors, such as seafood, garlic, and some cheeses, can be overwhelming and cause avoidance.
- **Unfamiliar fragrances:** New or unfamiliar fragrances can cause aversions and anxiety.

2. Observation and Documentation:

- **Reaction to Smell:** Pay attention to how the individual reacts to different food odors, taking note of any avoidance behaviors or bodily symptoms such as nausea.
- **Structured Exposure:** Gradually introduce foods with various odors in small amounts to pinpoint specific triggers. Document these events to have a full insight.

3. Engaging the Individual:

- **Sensitivity Discussions:** Discuss sensitivity to different odors and how it impacts their propensity to try new meals.
- **Comfort Level:** Make sure they are comfortable expressing their dislikes and concerns without fear of being judged.

Identifying Appearance Trigger

1. Common Appearance Sensitivities:

- **Color and Shape:** Unusual food colors or shapes may cause avoidance.
- **Presentation:** How food is presented (e.g., blended, special garnishes)

can also cause aversions.

2. Observation and Documentation:

- **Visual Reactions:** Note visual reactions to food, such as reluctance to touch or eat.
- **Controlled Exposure:** Present foods in a variety of ways and note which ones are more agreeable or cause discomfort.

3. Engaging the Individual:

- **Preference Inquiry:** Inquire about the individual's preferences for food appearance, such as color, shape, and presentation style.
- **Supportive Environment:** Provide a safe area for them to discuss their thoughts and feelings about food appearance without feeling judged.

Strategies for Managing Sensory Triggers

1. Gradual Exposure:

- **Small Steps:** To build tolerance over time, progressively introduce sensory triggers in little doses.
- **Pairing with Safe Foods:** Pairing unfamiliar or triggering foods with old and safe foods might help reduce anxiety and promote acceptance.

2. Sensory Desensitization:

- **Controlled Exposure Therapy:** Collaborate with a therapist to use controlled exposure therapy, progressively increasing exposure to sensory triggers in a supportive environment.
- **Positive Reinforcement:** Use positive reinforcement to boost progress and minimize negative associations with certain foods.

3. Customising Food Preparation:

- **Texture Modification:** To make foods more appealing, modify their texture by blending, pureeing, or changing cooking procedures.
- **Smell Management:** To reduce strong odors, cook foods in a well-ventilated location or start with lighter seasonings.
- **Appearance Adjustment:** Present foods in visually appealing ways that are appropriate for the individual's tastes, such as separating components or utilizing familiar forms and colors.

Exposure Therapy Techniques for Reducing Sensory Aversion

Exposure treatment is an effective method for reducing sensory aversion in people with Avoidant/Restrictive Food Intake Disorder (ARFID). This therapeutic technique gradually exposes people to feared foods in a controlled and supportive environment, allowing them to develop tolerance and lessen anxiety. Here are some realistic exposure therapy approaches for overcoming sensory aversions to texture, smell, and sight.

Understanding Exposure Therapy

1. Basics of Exposure Therapy:

- **Definition:** Exposure therapy is the gradual introduction of feared stimuli to diminish the associated anxiety over time.
- **Purpose:** For ARFID, the goal is to help individuals become more comfortable with foods they currently avoid due to sensory sensitivities.

2. Creating A Safe Environment:

- **Supportive Setting:** Make sure the therapy takes place in a peaceful and supportive environment where the patient feels safe.

- **Therapist Guidance:** Consult with a competent therapist who can guide the process, offer support, and alter exposure levels as necessary.

Gradual Exposure Techniques

1. Systematic Desensitisation:

- **Hierarchy of Fear:** Create a hierarchy of foods from least to most feared based on their sensory characteristics (texture, smell, appearance).
- **Step-by-Step Approach:** Begin with the least dreaded foods and progress to more demanding ones, allowing the individual to gain confidence and tolerance at each stage.

2. Incremental Exposure:

- **Take small steps:** Begin with extremely small amounts of the feared food, gradually increasing the amount over time.
- **Consistent Practice:** Schedule regular exposure sessions to increase familiarity and lessen fear. Being consistent is essential for making development.

Techniques to Reduce Texture Aversions

1. Texture Hierarchy:

- **Identify Textures:** Identify uncomfortable textures, such as crunchy, slimy, or mushy.
- **Gradual Introduction:** Start with textures that are slightly unpleasant yet workable.

2. Texture Modification:

- **Texture Modification:** Modify food texture to improve initial acceptability. For example, mix or puree foods to decrease their unpleasant properties.
- **Texture Gradation:** A gradual transition from modified textures to their original form. For example, go from pureed to mashed to solid versions of a specific dish.

Techniques to Reduce Smell Aversions

1. Controlled Smell Exposure:

- **Hierarchy of Smells:** Make a hierarchy of food odors, beginning with mild and progressing to stronger.
- **Gradual Smell Exposure:** Expose the individual to various food odors in a controlled manner, beginning with milder aromas and gradually increasing in intensity.

2. Desensitizing Smells:

- **Pairing with Pleasant Smells:** Pairing aversive aromas with pleasant or neutral smells might diminish negative associations.
- **Familiarisation:** Allow the individual to spend time in places with the smell without feeling compelled to eat the meal right away.

Techniques to Reduce Appearance Aversions

1. Visual Exposure:

- **Hierarchy of Appearances:** Create a hierarchy of food appearances, including color, shape, and presentation.
- **Incremental Visual Exposure:** Begin with showing the individual photographs of the item, then continue to examine the actual food, and finally

touch and taste it.

2. Presentation Adjustment:

- **Appealing Presentation:** Present foods in a visually pleasant and non-threatening manner. For example, arrange the food in recognizable shapes or add garnishes to make it look more appealing.
- **Gradual Introduction:** Gradually alter the appearance of food. Begin with minimal changes and gradually go to the original presentation.

Strategies for Safe Eating and Reducing Anxiety

The fear of choking is a major issue for many people suffering from Avoidant/Restrictive Food Intake Disorder. This anxiety might cause serious food avoidance and nutritional deficits. Understanding the source of this anxiety is critical for resolving it properly.

The Nature of Fear

1. Fear of Choking:

- **Definition:** The fear of choking is severe anxiety about the risk of food becoming caught in the throat, resulting in asphyxia or death.
- **Impact:** This anxiety may induce people to avoid particular textures or types of food, resulting in restrictive eating habits.

Psychological Underpinnings

1. Traumatic Experiences:

- **Past Choking Incidents:** Previous Choking Incidents A previous choking episode can be a strong motivator for establishing a fear of choking. The recollection of the event can form a long-lasting link between eating and risk.

- **Witnessing Choking:** Seeing someone else choke can inspire dread, particularly in young children who may not completely comprehend the situation but recognize the risk.

2. Anxiety Disorders:

- **General Anxiety:** People with a history of anxiety disorders may experience a fear of choking. Generalized anxiety can increase specific worries, increasing their intensity and persistence.
- **Health Anxiety:** Health-related anxiety, often known as hypochondria, can cause undue worry about choking, even when the risk is modest. This can lead to extreme caution or avoidance of specific meals.

3. Sensory Processing Issues:

- **Heightened Sensitivity:** Individuals with high sensory sensitivity may find the feeling of swallowing particular textures overwhelming, resulting in a panic response.
- **Texture Aversion:** Discomfort with certain textures can add to anxiety over swallowing, resulting in a fear of choking on particular textures.

Physical Factors

1. Medical Conditions:

- **Gastroesophageal Reflux Disease (GERD):** GERD can produce discomfort and the sense of food stuck in the throat, leading to worries of choking.
- **Swallowing Difficulties:** Physical swallowing difficulties, such as dysphagia, might increase the likelihood of choking and hence exacerbate the

dread.

2. Developmental Factors:

- **Young Children:** Children are inherently more prone to choking due to their smaller airways and developing feeding abilities. This susceptibility might lead to increased alertness and worry when eating.
- **Developmental Disorders:** Developmental disorders, such as autism spectrum disorder (ASD), can cause sensory sensitivities and anxiety, both of which can lead to a fear of choking.

Cognitive and Behavioural Aspects

1. Catastrophic Thinking:

- **Overestimation of Risk:** Individuals with ARFID may overestimate the risk and severity of choking. This catastrophic thinking might heighten the fear's intensity and threat.
- **Avoidance Behaviour:** Avoiding specific meals promotes fear. The more a person avoids feared foods, the stronger the link between them and risk gets.

2. Control Issues:

- **Need for Control:** The need for control can lead to rigid eating habits and avoidance of dangerous foods. This can result from underlying fear and a desire to reduce perceived threats.

Addressing the Fear

1. Therapeutic Interventions:

- **Cognitive Behavioral Therapy (CBT): CBT** can help individuals reframe their views about choking and lessen catastrophic thinking. It also includes ways of dealing with anxiety.
- **Exposure Therapy:** Gradual exposure to feared foods in a controlled and supportive setting can help people overcome their fears and gain confidence in their abilities to eat safely.

2. Medical Support:

- **Swallowing assessments:** A thorough evaluation by a speech-language pathologist can uncover any physical swallowing challenges and suggest treatment options.
- **Medical Management:** For disorders such as GERD, proper medical treatment can alleviate symptoms that lead to the fear of choking.

3. Sensory Integration Therapy:

- **Sensory Desensitisation:** Techniques to lessen sensory sensitivities can improve comfort with diverse food textures and reduce anxiety about swallowing.
- **Texture Gradual Introduction:** Gradually introducing different textures in a supportive manner can help increase tolerance and lessen fear.

Safe Swallowing Techniques and Modified Food Consistency

For people with ARFID, the fear of choking can be crippling, leading to extreme food avoidance. Implementing safe swallowing skills and adjusting food consistency can help alleviate these concerns and promote safer eating experiences.

Safe Swallowing Techniques

1. Chewing Thoroughly:

- **Importance:** Chewing thoroughly reduces the danger of choking by breaking down food into smaller pieces.
- **Practice:** Encourage eating small chunks and chewing them thoroughly before swallowing. Counting chews (e.g., 20 for each bite) can aid improve thoroughness.

2. Eating Slowly:

- **Important:** Eating slowly improves swallowing control and lowers the risk of choking.
- **Techniques:** Encourage mindful eating by emphasizing the sensory experience of food. Encourage putting down utensils between bites to help pace the meal.

3. Posture:

- **Importance:** Proper posture improves swallowing and prevents food from going the wrong way.
- **Advice:** Sit erect with a straight back and both feet on the ground. Keep the head slightly inclined forward to help with swallowing.

4. Small Sips of Liquids:

- **Important:** Taking small sips of liquids might aid in digestion and prevent throat irritation.
- **Tips:** Encourage alternating bits of food and sips of fluids. Avoid downing

huge volumes of fluids at once.

5. Controlled Breathing:

- **Importance:** Controlled breathing helps reduce anxiety and enhance focus during swallowing.
- **Practice:** Take a few deep breaths before beginning to eat. Continue to breathe gently and steadily throughout the meal.

Modified Food Consistency

1. Pureeing and Mashing:

- **Purpose:** Pureeing or mashing meals can make them simpler to swallow while maintaining nutritional content.
- **Application:** Use a blender or food processor to purée items into a smooth consistency. For softer foods, mashing with a fork may be sufficient.

2. Soft and Moist Foods:

- **Purpose:** Softer foods are simpler to swallow and reduce the risk of choking.
- **Examples:** Yogurt, applesauce, mashed potatoes, scrambled eggs, and well-cooked veggies are also suitable options.

3. Avoiding Dry and Hard Foods:

- **Purpose:** These foods are more likely to cause choking and make swallowing difficult.
- **Avoidance:** Avoid foods such as crackers, nuts, raw veggies, and rough meats. If these items must be eaten, they should be altered to a safer consistency.

4. Cutting and Slicing:

- **Purpose:** To lessen the danger of choking, cut foods into small, manageable pieces.
- **Techniques:** Cut all items into little, bite-sized pieces before eating. This is especially crucial with meats and fibrous veggies.

5. Thickeners for Liquids:

- **Purpose:** Adding thickeners helps slow down swallowing and lessen the danger of aspiration.
- **Products:** Commercial thickeners can be added to beverages to produce the required consistency. Thicker liquids, such as honey or nectar, should flow slower than water.

Implementing Safe Swallowing with Modified Consistency

1. Personalised assessment:

- **Professional evaluation:** A speech-language pathologist can conduct a swallowing exam to detect particular problems and offer appropriate solutions.
- **Individualized Plan:** Using the assessment, a personalized plan can be created to suit specific needs and ensure safe swallowing.

2. Gradual Transition:

- **Step-by-Step Approach:** Gradually introduce modified foods and safe swallowing techniques to allow the individual to adjust comfortably.
- **Monitor Progress:** Keep track of your progress and make adjustments as necessary. Regularly examine and revise the plan with professional assistance.

3. Practice and Reinforcements:

- **Consistent Practice:** Regularly practicing safe swallowing procedures might help you gain confidence and minimize anxiety.
- **Positive Reinforcement:** Encourage and recognize efforts to utilize safe swallowing procedures. Celebrate minor accomplishments to keep yourself motivated.

4.Supportive Environment:

- **Encouragement:** Create a friendly dining atmosphere where individuals feel safe and encouraged to try new ways.
- **Family Involvement:** Educate family members on safe swallowing techniques and dietary changes to provide ongoing help at home.

Cognitive Behavioral Therapy for Managing Anxiety Around Choking

Cognitive Behavioural Therapy (CBT) is a highly effective treatment for controlling choking anxiety in people with ARFID. CBT focuses on recognizing and modifying harmful thought patterns and behaviors to help people establish healthy coping mechanisms and overcome their fear of choking.

Understanding CBT

1. Cognitive component:

- **Thought Patterns:** CBT teaches people how to recognize and challenge unreasonable or exaggerated choking thoughts. For example, the belief that "I will choke every time I eat" is addressed and replaced with more realistic thoughts.
- **Cognitive Restructuring:** This strategy entails challenging the facts

supporting frightening thoughts and replacing them with more balanced and correct beliefs.

2. Behavioural Component:

- **Behavioral Experiments:** Individuals are advised to test their frightened choking predictions safely and gradually. This helps children realize that their anxieties are generally unwarranted.
- **Exposure Therapy:** Gradual exposure to feared foods and eating settings helps people desensitize their anxiety, resulting in fewer avoidance behaviors over time.

Implementing CBT for Choking Anxiety

1. Identifying Triggers:

- **Awareness:** The first stage in CBT is identifying specific triggers that create worry about choking. These can include specific meals, textures, or eating situations.
- **Recording Triggers:** Keeping a journal of situations and foods that cause anxiety might help individuals and therapists better recognize patterns and tailor treatment.

2. Cognitive Restructuring:

- **Challenging Negative Thoughts:** Cognitive restructuring involves challenging negative attitudes about choking. For example, the idea "I will choke on this food" can be challenged and replaced by "I have eaten this food many times without choking."
- **Evidence-Based Thinking:** Encouraging people to seek out evidence that contradicts their anxieties will help them build a more balanced

perspective.

3. Gradual Exposure:

- **Hierarchy of Fears:** Creating a hierarchy of feared foods and events, from least to most anxiety-provoking, promotes gradual exposure.
- **Controlled Exposure:** Beginning with less dreaded foods or lesser portions, people gradually confront their concerns in a safe and supportive atmosphere.
- **Repetitive Practice:** Regular and repetitive exposure helps to desensitize the individual to the fear of choking, hence increasing confidence with time.

4. Relaxation Techniques:

- **Breathing Exercises:** Deep breathing and relaxation exercises can alleviate physiological symptoms of anxiety, including rapid heartbeat and shallow breathing.
- **Mindfulness:** Mindfulness activities, such as focusing on the present moment and eating deliberately, can help to reduce anxiety and improve relaxation during meals.

5. Behavioural Experiments:

- **Testing Predictions:** Individuals can test their frightened predictions in a safe and controlled setting. For example, taking a little bite of a feared food and witnessing the reaction can assist refute unjustified phobias.
- **Recording Outcomes:** Keeping track of the results of these experiments reinforces the idea that choking is less prevalent than previously thought.

Expanding Your Repertoire: Building a More Varied Diet

Individuals with ARFID may rely on a very narrow selection of "safe" foods due to food-related fear and anxiety. While eating these foods may alleviate anxiety in the short term, this habit, known as the "safe food trap," can pose serious threats to one's health and well-being.

The Appeal of Safe Food

1. Anxiety Reduction:

- **Predictability:** Safe meals are recognizable and predictable, which can considerably lessen anxiety about eating.
- **Comfort:** These foods are frequently associated with happy experiences, making them appealing options.

2. Sense of Control:

- **Control Over Eating:** Safe meals can provide a sense of control during stressful situations. Knowing that food is "safe" can help to reduce stress during meals.
- **Avoidance of Fear:** By sticking to safe foods, people can avoid the anxiety and discomfort that comes with trying new or feared foods.

Risks of the Safe Food Trap

1. Nutritional Deficiencies:

- **Limited Nutrient consumption:** Relying on a limited variety of foods can lead to insufficient consumption of important nutrients. Each food group contains certain vitamins, minerals, and macronutrients required for health.

- **Health Effects:** Nutritional deficiencies can cause a variety of health problems, including decreased immunity, poor bone health, anemia, and cognitive impairment.

2. Physical Health Decline:

- **Growth and Development:** Limited diets can impede growth and development in children and adolescents, resulting in stunting, developmental delays, and other health concerns.
- **Chronic Conditions:** Nutritional shortages and imbalanced diets can lead to long-term health problems like osteoporosis, heart disease, and diabetes.

3. Social and Emotional Impact:

- **Social Isolation:** Sticking to safe foods might lead to avoiding social events with food, such as parties, family gatherings, and dining out. This isolation can worsen emotions of loneliness and sadness.
- **Emotional Stress:** Constantly worrying about having access to healthy foods can cause severe emotional stress and anxiety, reducing overall quality of life.

4. Reinforcement of dread:

- **Avoidance Behaviour:** Consistently avoiding unsafe foods strengthens the related dread and anxiety. This avoidance makes it more difficult to broaden the diet in the future.
- **Increased Anxiety:** The longer a person follows a restricted diet, the more ingrained their anxiety and dread of new foods grow, resulting in a vicious cycle.

Breaking Free of the Safe Food Trap

1. Gradual Introduction of New Foods:

- **Small Steps:** Introduce new foods gradually, taking little steps. Introduce new meals carefully and in tiny quantities. Combining new foods with safe foods can help make the process less intimidating.
- **Positive Reinforcement:** Celebrate little triumphs and progress towards trying new meals. Positive reinforcement can help people gain confidence and lessen anxiety.

2. Exposure Therapy:

- **Controlled Exposure:** Controlled exposure to unfamiliar meals in a supportive atmosphere can help reduce fear. Begin with less anxiety-inducing foods and then proceed to more problematic ones.
- **Consistency:** Regular exposure and practice are essential for lowering apprehension and increasing familiarity with new foods.

3. Professional Support:

- **Therapists and dietitians:** Working with a therapist and a trained dietitian can provide the necessary guidance and support for safely expanding one's diet. Therapists can help with underlying anxiety, and nutritionists can ensure dietary demands are addressed.
- **Personalized Plans:** Create personalized meal plans with a variety of foods to guarantee balanced nutrition. Tailoring strategies to individual preferences and tolerances might help make the process more doable.

4. Mindfulness and relaxation:

- **Mindful eating:** Mindful eating can help people focus on their sensory experiences while eating, reducing anxiety and creating a healthy relationship with food.

- **Relaxation Techniques:** Deep breathing and progressive muscle relaxation are two relaxation techniques that can help people control their anxiety during eating.

Introducing New Foods Through Pairing and Positive Reinforcement

For those with ARFID, introducing new foods can be difficult and anxiety-inducing. However, tactics such as mixing new foods with familiar ones and utilizing positive reinforcement can help make the transition easier and more successful.

The Pairing Strategy

1. Pairing with safe foods:

- **Familiarity:** Combining novel foods with safe, familiar ones might help alleviate anxiety by creating a sense of comfort and predictability.
- **Taste Masking:** Using a favorite meal's flavor to disguise the taste of a new cuisine might make it more appealing and less terrifying.

2. Gradual Integration:

- **Small Portions:** Introduce new food in tiny portions alongside existing safe foods. This can make the unfamiliar cuisine appear less intimidating.
- **Incremental Increase:** As you become more comfortable with the new cuisine, gradually increase your intake.

3. Blending and Mixing:

- **Blending Foods:** Incorporate new foods into familiar recipes by adding veggies to a smoothie or a small amount of a new item to a favorite casserole.
- **Layering:** Combine new and safe foods in a way that blends them seamlessly, such as adding a little piece of a new fruit to yogurt.

4. Sensory Gradation:

- **Texture and Appearance:** Adjust the new food's texture and look to match safe items. For example, if the individual loves pureed foods, begin with a pureed version of the new dish and gradually transition to more solid versions.

Using Positive Reinforcement

1. Celebrating Small Wins:

- **Acknowledgement:** Recognize and celebrate each step forward, no matter how small. This could be as simple as tasting a new food or taking a small bite.
- **Rewards:** Use a reward system to encourage trying new foods. Rewards can be non-food related, such as extra playtime, a favorite activity, or a small toy.

2. Encouragement and Praise:

- **Positive Feedback:** Use consistent, positive feedback to reinforce improvement. Comments like "You did great trying that new food!" can enhance self-esteem and motivation.
- **Supportive atmosphere:** Make sure the dining atmosphere is positive and pressure-free. If the individual is hesitant, refrain from making nasty comments or expressing irritation.

3.Visual Progress Tracking:

- **Charts and Stickers:** To track accomplishment, use visual aids such as progress charts or sticker systems. Seeing actual results may be both motivating and satisfying.
- **Goal Setting:** Set realistic goals for sampling new foods and celebrate when they are met.

4. Involving Individuals:

- **Choice and Control:** Allow the individual to have some say in the process by allowing them to choose which new items to sample and how they are cooked.
- **Participation:** Involve them in food preparation. Cooking or meal preparation can help to boost interest in new meals while decreasing anxiety.

Practical Steps to Implementation

1. Begin Simple:

- **Mild Flavours:** Begin by introducing new meals that have mild flavors and are similar to previously acceptable items. This lowers the probability of severe adverse responses.
- **Consistent Routine:** To increase familiarity, incorporate new foods into your routine on a regular basis. Consistency helps to eliminate unpredictability, which can induce anxiety.

2. Sensory Exploration:

- **Non-Eating Activities:** Allow for exploration of new foods outside of mealtimes. Touching, smelling, and playing with food can help develop comfort without the need to eat.

- **Desensitization:** Gradual exposure to the look, smell, and texture of novel foods can make the tasting and eating experience less daunting.

3. Professional Support:

- **Therapeutic guidance:** Collaborate with therapists and nutritionists who can offer structured and personalized help. They are effective in guiding the usage of pairing and positive reinforcement approaches.
- **Individualized plans:** Customise techniques to meet the individual's personal demands and preferences. What works for one individual might not work for another, therefore personalization is essential.

Setting Realistic Goals and Celebrating Small Victories

When striving to overcome ARFID, it is critical to set realistic goals and celebrate little successes. This method promotes motivation, and confidence, and makes the transition to a more diverse and nutritious diet more easy and enjoyable.

Setting Realistic Goals

1. Understand the baseline:

- **Current intake:** Begin by noting the individual's existing dietary preferences. This provides a basis from which to create attainable goals.
- **Identify challenges:** Understand the individual obstacles and worries associated with new foods, such as texture, taste, and color.

2. SMART goals:

- **Specific:** Set clear and explicit goals. For example, "Try a new vegetable once a week" works better than "Eat more vegetables."

- **Measurable:** Make sure your goals are measurable. This facilitates tracking progress and celebrating accomplishments. For example, "take two bites of a new fruit" is a clear indicator of accomplishment.
- **Achievable:** Goals should be practical and achievable. Begin with gradual, reasonable modifications to prevent overwhelming the individual.
- **Relevant:** Set significant and relevant goals for the individual's overall improvement. Focus on introducing foods that can increase nutritional diversity.
- **Time-bound:** Determine a timeline for completing each goal. This offers structure and helps you stay focused. For example, "Introduce one new food by the end of the month."

3. Incremental Progress:

- **Step-by-Step Approach:** Break down larger ambitions into smaller, gradual actions. For example, if the goal is to eat a new sort of fruit, start by looking at it, then touching it, and lastly tasting it.
- **Gradual Increase:** Gradually increase the difficulty of your aims. Begin with less scary dishes and gradually introduce more difficult ones.

4. Flexibility:

- **Adjustable goals:** Be adaptable and open to change goals based on the individual's comfort and development. If a goal seems too difficult, break it down further or take a step back and attempt a different strategy.
- **Personalized goals:** Tailor goals to the individual's specific requirements and interests. What works for one individual may not work for others.

Celebrating small victories

1. Acknowledge Progress:

- **Recognition:** Recognize and applaud every step forward, no matter how tiny. Recognizing progress encourages positive behavior and increases confidence.
- **Positive Feedback:** Give continuous positive feedback. Words like "Great job trying that new food!" or "I'm proud of you for taking a bite!" can increase morale and motivation.

2. Reward Systems:

- **Non-Food Rewards:** Use non-food prizes to recognize accomplishments. Extra playtime, a favorite pastime, stickers, or a little toy are all possible rewards.
- **Immediate prizes:** Give prizes right away after completing a task to reinforce the link between the behavior and the reward.

3. Visual Tracking:

- **Progress Charts:** Use charts or stickers to track progress. This creates a concrete depiction of accomplishments and can be quite motivating.
- **Milestone Markers:** Place major milestones on the chart and celebrate when they are met. This promotes a sense of accomplishment and growth.

4. Emotional Support:

- **Encouragement:** Provide ongoing encouragement and support. A friendly and supportive environment reduces stress and makes the procedure more fun.
- **Celebrate together:** Involve family and friends in victory celebrations.

Shared celebrations can boost motivation and provide extra encouragement.

5. Reflect and Reinforce:

- **Reflection:** Take time to reflect on your progress. Discuss what techniques were effective and what should be improved.
- **Reinforcement:** Reinforce effective strategies and build on them. Consistent reinforcement promotes momentum and progress.

Practical Steps to Implementation

1. Start small:

- **Initial Steps:** Start with extremely tiny, manageable goals. For example, touching or smelling a new meal can be a pre-tasting stage.
- **Incremental challenges:** As you become more comfortable, gradually increase the level of difficulty. Move from touching and smelling to tasting and then swallowing greater portions.

2. Involvement and Choice:

- **Active Participation:** Involve the individual in defining goals and selecting incentives. This reinforces their sense of control and devotion.
- **Empowerment:** Allow them to choose which new foods to eat and how to incorporate them into meals.

3. Regular Review:

- **Progress Check-ins:** Regularly assess and change goals in response to progress and criticism. Celebrate your accomplishments and set new, somewhat more demanding goals.

- **Therapist and Dietitian Support:** Collaborate with therapists and nutritionists to establish realistic goals and build successful solutions. Their experience can help guide the procedure and ensure that nutritional requirements are met.

7

Chapter 7: Building Resilience and Empowerment on Your ARFID Journey

Mindfulness and Relaxation Techniques for Managing Anxiety

Mindfulness activities can be quite useful in stress management and emotional eating reduction, particularly for people who have ARFID. Mindfulness can help interrupt the cycle of stress and emotional responses to food by focusing on the present moment and creating a nonjudgmental awareness of thoughts and feelings.

Understanding Mindfulness

Mindfulness is the practice of paying attention to the present moment without judgment. It promotes awareness of thoughts, emotions, physiological sensations, and the surroundings. This practice can help people recognize and respond to their needs and emotions healthily and constructively.

Techniques for mindfulness

1. Mindful Breathing:

- **Focus on the Breath:** Sit comfortably and concentrate on your breath. Consider the sensation of air entering and exiting your nostrils, the rise and fall of your chest, and the rhythm of your breathing.
- **Counting Breaths:** Count each breath up to ten, then start again. This helps to focus your attention and quiet the mind.
- **Deep Breathing:** Inhale slowly through the nose, hold for a few seconds, and then exhale slowly through the mouth. Deep breathing can help relieve anxiety and increase calm.

2. Body Scan:

- **Progressive Awareness:** Focus on each part of your body, beginning with your toes and progressing to your head. Recognize any tension, discomfort, or symptoms without attempting to change them.
- **Relaxation:** As you become more aware of each body part, intentionally release any tension you notice. This technique encourages calm and a greater connection to your body.

3. Mindful Eating:

- **Slow down:** Eat slowly and thoughtfully, focusing on the flavor, texture, and scent of each bite. Chew thoroughly and enjoy the sensation.
- **Avoid Distractions:** Don't eat while watching TV, using your phone, or working. Concentrate entirely on the act of eating.
- **Gratitude:** Before you eat, take a moment to enjoy the meal, thinking about where it came from and how much effort it took to prepare.

4. Mindful Meditation:

- **Guided Meditations:** Try guided meditation apps or CDs emphasizing mindfulness. These might add structure and support to your practice.
- **Quiet Space:** Locate a quiet, comfortable area where you will not be bothered. Sit or lie in a relaxed stance.
- **Focus and Redirect:** When your mind wanders, softly return your attention to your breath or the guided directions without judgment.

5. Journaling:

- **Reflective Writing:** Spend a few minutes daily jotting down your ideas and feelings. This can help you digest your emotions and identify trends in your eating habits.
- **Gratitude Journal:** Keep a journal in which you record the things you are grateful for. This can shift the attention away from stress and negativity, fostering a more optimistic view.

Applying Mindfulness to Reduce Emotional Eating

1. Recognise emotional triggers:

- **Identify Triggers:** Pay attention to situations, ideas, or feelings that make you want to eat. Recognizing these triggers is the first step towards managing them consciously.
- **Pause and Reflect:** Before grabbing food, ask yourself if you are hungry or if you are eating to deal with your emotions. Consider how you are feeling and why.

2. Establish a Mindful Eating Environment:

- **Set the scene:** Create a relaxing and enjoyable eating environment. Set the table, remove any distractions, and concentrate on the food.
- **Eat with purpose:** Approach every meal to nourish your body. This

mentality shift has the potential to help reduce emotional eating.

3. Develop alternative coping strategies:

- **Mindful Activities:** Walking, yoga, or listening to relaxing music are all examples of mindfulness and relaxation-promoting activities.
- **Emotional Support:** When feeling overwhelmed, seek help from friends, family, or a therapist. Talking about your feelings can help you feel better and lessen your emotional eating.

4. Practice self-compassion:

- **Be kind to yourself:** Treat yourself with compassion and understanding, especially during stressful times. Recognize that it is acceptable to have setbacks and that improvement takes time.
- **Positive Affirmations:** Use positive affirmations to strengthen your caring thinking. Remind yourself of your qualities and abilities.

5. Establish a Routine:

- **Consistent Practice:** Include mindfulness practices in your daily routine. Consistency makes mindfulness a natural part of your life, increasing its advantages.
- **Scheduled Meals:** Set regular meal times to reduce impulsive eating. A regimen can provide structure while also reducing stress associated with eating.

Deep Breathing Exercises and Relaxation Techniques

Deep breathing exercises and relaxation techniques are critical tools for dealing with the stress, anxiety, and emotional issues connected with ARFID. These activities assist in quieting the mind, relax the body, and promote a sense of well-being, making them important components of a complete approach to therapy and rehabilitation.

1. Deep breathing exercises

- **Position:** Sit or lie down in a comfortable position. Place one hand on your chest, and the other on your abdomen.
- **Inhale:** Take a slow breath through your nose, allowing your abdomen to rise as you fill your lungs with air. Your chest should be reasonably motionless.
- **Exhale:** Exhale slowly through your mouth, allowing your abdomen to fall. Concentrate on the sensation of your breathing and the movement of your abdomen.
- **Repeat:** Continue this breathing pattern for 5-10 minutes, taking slow, deep breaths.

2. 4-7-8 Breathing:

- **Position:** Sit or lay down in a comfortable position.
- **Inhale:** Close your eyes and breathe quietly through your nose for a count of four.
- **Hold:** Hold your breath for the count of seven.
- **Exhale:** Exhale entirely through your mouth, generating a whooshing sound, for a count of eight.
- **Repeat:** Repeat the cycle four times first, then increase to eight as you grow more comfortable.

3. Box Breathing (Square Breathing):

- **Position:** Sit comfortably with your feet flat on the ground and your hands in your lap.
- **Inhale:** Take a four-count breath through your nose.
- **Hold:** Hold your breath for the count of four.
- **Exhale:** Breathe out through your mouth for four counts.

- **Hold:** Hold your breath for the count of four.
- **Repeat:** Repeat the procedure for several minutes, visualizing a square with each inhalation.

4. Alternate nostril breathing (Nadi Shodhana):

- **Position:** Sit in a comfortable position, spine straight.
- **Close Right Nostril:** Use your right thumb to close the right nostril. Inhale deeply from the left nostril.
- **Switch:** Close your left nostril with your right ring finger and then release your right nose. Exhale from your right nostril.
- **Inhale Right Nostril:** Inhale deeply from the right nostril.
- **Switch:** Close your right nostril with your right thumb and then open your left nostril. Exhale from your left nostril.
- **Repeat:** Repeat this pattern for a few minutes, concentrating on your breath and the sensation of air going through your nose.

Relaxation Techniques

1. Progressive Muscular Relaxation (PMR):

- **Tense and Relax:** Starting at your toes and working your way up to your head, tense each muscle group for 5-10 seconds before releasing. Concentrate on the difference between stress and relaxation.
- **Sequence:** Follow this order: toes, feet, calves, thighs, abdomen, chest, hands, arms, shoulders, neck, and face.
- **Breathe:** Breathe in as you tense your muscles, and exhale as you relax.

2. Visualization:

- **Find a Quiet Space:** Sit or lie down in a calm, pleasant environment.
- **Create a scene:** Close your eyes and envision a tranquil setting, such as

a beach, forest, or meadow. Use all of your senses to make the scene as vivid as possible.

- **Relax:** Take a few minutes to relax and absorb the imagery, focusing on the nuances and sensations of the scenario.

3. Guided Imagery:

- **Audio Guides:** Use audio guides or applications to calmly visualize and experience scenes.
- **Personal Visualisation:** Alternatively, you can develop your mental imagery based on places or events that bring you comfort and calm.

4. Mindful Meditation:

- **Focus on Breath:** Sit comfortably and concentrate on your breath. Observe the feelings of breathing without trying to change them.
- **Body Scan:** Mentally scan your body from head to toe, noting any points of tension or discomfort.
- **Nonjudgmental Awareness:** Recognise thoughts and feelings as they arise and let them pass without judgment. Gently return your concentration to your breath or body scan.

5. Yoga and Stretching:

- **Gentle Yoga:** Practice easy yoga poses and stretches to increase relaxation and flexibility. Concentrate on deep breathing and deliberate movement.
- **Stretching program:** Use a regular stretching program that targets main muscle groups to relieve stress and enhance circulation.

Building Body Positivity and Self-Compassion

Negative body image beliefs can be a significant challenge for those with ARFID, leading to feelings of inadequacy and low self-esteem. Challenging these thoughts is critical to developing a healthier relationship with one's body and boosting general well-being. Here are some practical ways to challenge and modify negative body image thoughts:

Understanding Negative Body Image Thoughts.

Negative body image beliefs are frequently rooted in unrealistic ideals and critical self-perception. These thoughts can be persistent and harmful, affecting mental health and daily function. Recognizing and addressing these attitudes is the first step in developing a good body image.

Strategies for Addressing Negative Body Image Thoughts

1. Identify and Acknowledge Negative Thoughts:

- **Awareness:** Pay attention to the times when you have negative ideas about your physique. Write them down to identify patterns and triggers.
- **Name the Thoughts:** Label these thoughts as "negative body image thoughts" to isolate them and weaken their influence.

2. Question the Validity of Negative Thoughts:

- **Evidence Check:** Ask yourself two questions: "What evidence do I have that supports this thought?" Additionally, "What evidence do I have that contradicts it?" This helps to identify the irrationality of many negative attitudes.
- **Alternative Perspective:** Consider how a compassionate friend would perceive the issue. Would they agree with your negative evaluation or

provide a more positive perspective?

3. reframe negative thoughts:

- **Positive Reframe:** Replace negative thoughts with affirmative or neutral statements. For example, instead of saying "I hate my body," say "My body is capable and deserves care."
- **Focus on functionality:** Focus on what your body is capable of rather than how it seems. Recognize your body's capabilities and strengths.

4. Practice Self-Compassion:

- **Kindness:** Treat yourself with care and understanding, just as you would a friend. Recognize that everyone has flaws and that outward looks do not determine self-worth.
- **Self-Compassion Exercises:** Try exercises that encourage self-compassion, such as writing a letter to yourself from the perspective of a supportive friend.

5. Challenge Societal Standards:

- **Media literacy:** Be skeptical of media messaging and cultural ideals of beauty. Recognize that many photographs have been manipulated and do not accurately depict reality.
- **Diverse Representation:** Look for and support media that encourages diverse and realistic portrayals of bodies.

6. Surround yourself with positivity:

- **Supportive People:** Spend time with people who are pleasant and encouraging, and who value you for who you are rather than your appearance.
- **Positive Influences:** Follow social media accounts and interact with information that encourages body positivity and self-acceptance.

7. Create Healthy Habits:

- **Nourishing Activities:** Enjoy things that make you feel good about your body, including exercise, dance, or yoga. Consider how these activities make you feel rather than how they may affect your appearance.
- **Self-Care:** Establish self-care practices that will make you feel loved and valued. This can involve skincare, wearing comfy clothes, and engaging in hobbies that you enjoy.

8. Set Realistic Goals:

- **Realistic Expectations:** Set realistic goals for body image and self-esteem. Celebrate modest successes and development instead of striving for perfection.
- **Personal Growth:** Prioritise personal development and accomplishments that are unrelated to looks. Building skills, pursuing hobbies, and attaining goals can all help build self-esteem.

Practicing Self-Acceptance and Self-Love

Practicing self-acceptance and self-love is critical for those coping with ARFID since it helps to lay a solid basis for recovery and overall health. These practices entail accepting who you are, acknowledging your intrinsic worth, and treating yourself with care and compassion.

Understanding Self-Acceptance and Love

Self-acceptance entails recognizing and accepting all aspects of oneself, including both strengths and weaknesses. It entails accepting your emotions, thoughts, and experiences without judgment.

Self-love is defined as being loving and compassionate to oneself. It entails caring for your physical, emotional, and mental well, as well as treating yourself with the same respect and care that you would give to someone you love.

Strategies to Practice Self-Acceptance and Self-Love

1. Recognise Your Worth:

- **Affirmations:** Use positive affirmations to emphasize your value. Phrases like "I am enough," "I deserve love and respect," and "I value myself" can be extremely effective.
- **Self-Reflection:** Take time to consider your accomplishments, characteristics, and unique contributions. Writing things down can help to strengthen your sense of self-worth.

2. Embrace Imperfections:

- **Recognize Humanity:** Realise that everyone has flaws and makes mistakes. Imperfections are part of what defines us as humans.
- **Self-forgiveness:** Learn to forgive yourself for previous mistakes and accept that they do not determine your worth.

3. Develop a Compassionate Inner Voice:

- **Positive self-talk:** Replace self-critical ideas with kind and encouraging self-talk. When you see yourself becoming self-critical, recast the concept in a more positive perspective.
- **Inner Dialogue:** Imagine speaking to yourself as you would to a close friend. Give yourself the same care and understanding.

4. Set Realistic Expectations:

- **Goals:** Create reasonable and achievable goals for yourself. Celebrate modest successes and development instead of striving for perfection.

- **Self-Patience:** Be patient with yourself while working towards your goals. Understand that progress requires time and effort.

5. Practice Self-Care:

- **Physical Care:** Exercise regularly, eat well, and get enough rest. Listen to your body's requirements and respond gently.
- **Emotional Care:** Engage in things that make you happy and relaxed. This could involve hobbies, spending time with loved ones, or practicing mindfulness.

6. Surround Yourself with Positivity:

- **Supportive Relationships:** Surround yourself with positivity through supportive relationships. Limit your interactions with those that deplete your energy or bring you down.
- **Positive Environment:** Create a living and working environment that encourages optimism and well-being. This could include decorating with your favorite items or organizing your area to alleviate stress.

7. Practice Gratitude:

- **Gratitude Journaling:** Keep a gratitude diary to periodically jot down things you are glad for. This technique might help you change your attention from what is missing to what is abundant in your life.
- **Mindful Appreciation:** Take time throughout the day to enjoy the little things, such as a gorgeous sunset, a nice gesture, or a personal accomplishment.

8. Seek Professional Support:

- **Therapy:** Therapy can help you overcome self-acceptance issues. Therapists can provide skills and approaches for developing self-love.

- **Support groups:** Joining support groups can provide a sense of community and shared understanding, allowing you to feel less alone on your path.

9. Use Mindfulness Practices:

- **Mindfulness Meditation:** Mindfulness meditation can help you become more aware of your thoughts and feelings without judgment. This can help you form a more empathetic relationship with yourself.
- **Body Scan:** Try a body scan meditation to reconnect with and appreciate your body. Identify any points of tension and breathe into them with warmth and tenderness.

Activities to Promote Self-Acceptance and Love

1. Write a Self-Compassion Letter:

- **Purpose:** Write yourself a letter of compassion, understanding, and support. Focus on areas where you struggle with self-acceptance and offer encouraging and loving words.

2. Create a Self-Love Ritual:

- **Routine:** Create a daily or weekly ritual for self-care. This could be taking a relaxing bath, going for a nature walk, or setting aside time for reading and thought.

3. Practice Mirror Work:

- **Affirmations:** Stand in front of a mirror and examine your eyes. Say positive affirmations aloud to reinforce your worth and beauty. This practice can help you develop a positive self-image.

4. Create a Gratitude Jar:

- **Daily Notes:** Write down what you are grateful for on small pieces of paper and save them in a jar. The jar will gradually fill with memories of positive elements of your life, which you may review whenever you need a lift.

5. Engage in Creative Expression:

- **Art and Writing:** Express yourself creatively through art or writing to explore your identity and emotions. Creative hobbies can be both healing and affirming.

Celebrating Milestones: Recognizing Your Progress on the Road to Recovery

Recognizing and applauding your accomplishments is a vital component of the ARFID rehabilitation process. It promotes self-esteem, reinforces positive behavior, and offers drive to keep moving forward.

Why Tracking Achievements is Important

Tracking your successes has various advantages:

- **Boosts Confidence:** Seeing your improvement increases your self-esteem and confidence.
- **Provides motivation:** Celebrating minor accomplishments helps you stay motivated and focused on your goals.
- **Reinforces Positive Behavior:** Recognizing your accomplishments motivates you to continue engaging in healthy behaviors.
- **Provides Perspective:** It allows you to recognize how far you've come, especially during difficult times.

Strategies for Identifying and Tracking Achievements.

1. Establish clear and realistic goals:

- **Specific Goals:** Set defined, achievable goals for your ARFID journey. Consider "Try a new food" or "Attend a social meal."
- **Short-Term and Long-Term Goals:** Create a balance of short-term goals that are readily accomplished and long-term goals that demand more time and effort.

2. Keep a daily or weekly journal:

- **Record Your Progress:** Keep a notebook of your successes every day or week. This could entail sampling new cuisines, overcoming anxiety during meals, or attending social gatherings.
- **Reflect:** Take time to reflect on your accomplishments and how they make you feel. Reflecting helps to reinforce positive experiences.

3. Use a Visual Tracker:

- **Charts and Graphics:** Make charts or graphs to graphically track your progress. This may include a dietary exposure chart in which you tick down new foods you've eaten, or a mood tracker to measure your emotional well-being progress.
- **Bullet diary:** Keep a bullet diary with sections for documenting objectives and successes. Include emblems or stickers to boost visual appeal and incentive.

4. Celebrate Small Victories:

- **Acknowledge Achievements:** Celebrate small victories and acknowledge achievements. Every step forward, no matter how minor, should be acknowledged. This could be as basic as finishing a meal or taking a mouthful of something new.

- **Rewards:** Treat yourself to little prizes for reaching your goals. Rewards can include non-food items such as a new book, a soothing bath, or a fun outing.

5. Share Your Successes:

- **With Loved Ones:** Share your achievements with family and friends who support you. Their encouragement and praise can help improve your motivation.
- **Support Groups:** Join support groups where you may share your progress and learn about other people's achievements. This promotes a sense of community and common purpose.

6. Establish a "Success Jar" or "Accomplishment Board":

- **Success Jar:** Record each success on a piece of paper and save it in a jar. Over time, you'll have a concrete record of your accomplishments to reflect on.
- **Accomplishment Board:** Create an Accomplishment Board on which you can pin or write about your accomplishments. This might include a bulletin board, a wall in your room, or a digital board.

7. Reflect on Growth During Setbacks:

- **Learn from Challenges:** When you suffer setbacks, think about what you've learned and how you might use this experience to improve.
- **Focus on Effort:** Recognise the effort you put in, even if the outcome was not what you expected. Effort and perseverance are inherently rewarding.

Practical Tools for Tracking Achievements

1. Apps and Digital Tools:

- **Habit-Tracking Apps:** Use habit-tracking applications to record daily achievements and monitor progress over time. Examples are Habitica, HabitBull, and Done.
- **Gratitude Apps:** Apps like Gratitude Journal and 5 Minute Journal can help you keep track of your everyday achievements and happy experiences.

2. Printed Planners and Journals:

- **Dedicated Journals:** Purchase a journal designed exclusively for charting your ARFID recovery experience. Look for ones that include prompts and areas for goal setting and reflection.
- **Planner Inserts:** Use planner inserts specifically developed for goal tracking and accomplishment journaling. These can be added to your current planner or notepad.

3. DIY Tools:

- **Create customized charts:** Create bespoke charts or templates to meet your individual needs and preferences. For easy design, use applications like Excel or Canva.
- **Scrapbook:** Keep a scrapbook of images, notes, and souvenirs that represent your achievements. This can be a fun and innovative approach to track progress.

Examples of Trackable Achievements

1. Food-related achievements:

- **Trying new foods:** Keep a record of every new cuisine you eat and your experiences with it.
- **Expanding Portions:** Keep track of your success as you increase your portion sizes or try new meals.
- **Eating in Social Settings:** Keep track of times you successfully eat in social situations or join others for meals.

2. Emotional and psychological milestones:

- **Managing Anxiety:** Keep track of times when you successfully manage anxiety during meals or other food-related circumstances.
- **Coping methods:** Monitor the usage and effectiveness of coping methods in managing ARFID symptoms.
- **Positive Self-Talk:** Make a note of moments when you effectively fought negative thoughts or used positive self-talk.

3. Social and functional enhancements:

- **Social Engagement:** Keep track of the social activities you engaged in, particularly those that involved eating.
- **Daily Routine:** Monitor progress in everyday routines, such as consistent meal times or successful meal preparation.
- **Physical Health:** Take note of any physical health changes, such as increased energy, weight stability, or better nutrient intake.

Rewarding Yourself for Reaching Goals

Rewarding oneself for meeting goals is an important aspect of keeping motivated and enjoying your progress toward conquering ARFID. Rewards not only provide positive reinforcement, but they also foster a sense of achievement and joy.

The Importance of Rewards for Recovery

Rewards are important in the rehabilitation process for a variety of reasons.

- **Encouragement:** Rewards motivate you to continue working towards your goals by giving you something to look forward to.
- **Positive Reinforcement:** They encourage positive behaviors and aid in the development of new, healthy habits.
- **Motivation:** Knowing there will be a reward at the end of your endeavor can improve motivation and make difficult jobs seem more feasible.
- **Self-Care:** Rewards can also be used to promote self-care by reminding you to nurture and love yourself.

How To Choose Effective Rewards

When selecting rewards, it is critical to choose items that are meaningful, fun, and nutritious. Below are some guidelines to consider:

1. Personal Significance:

- **Meaningful prizes:** Choose prizes with personal importance and joy. This could be something you've been meaning to accomplish or a treat you've been looking forward to.
- **Alignment with Values:** Ensure that the rewards are consistent with your values and contribute to your general well-being.

2. Non-food related:

- **Avoid food rewards:** To preserve a healthy relationship with eating, select non-food rewards. This focuses the attention on positive experiences rather than utilizing food as a reward.

3. Variety: Mix it up:

- **Mix It Up:** Use a range of incentives to keep things interesting. This could include experiences, tangible goods, or personal treats.
- **Small and Large Rewards:** Create a balance between tiny, immediate rewards for short-term goals and larger, more meaningful rewards for long-term accomplishments.

Examples of Reward Ideas

1. Experiences:

- **Day Trips:** Organize a day excursion to a favorite destination, like a beach, park, or museum.
- **Classes:** Enrol in a class that interests you, such as painting, cooking, or dance.
- **Entertainment:** Treat yourself to a movie night, concert, theatrical play, or sporting event.

2. Self-Care:

- **Spa Day:** Plan a spa day with massages, facials, or other calming treatments.
- **Relaxation:** Take a day to indulge in your favorite soothing hobbies, such as reading a book, taking a long bath, or meditation.
- **Fitness:** Sign up for a fitness class that you've always wanted to take, such

as yoga, pilates, or dancing.

3. Hobbies and Interests:

- **New supplies:** Purchase new hobby items, such as art materials, gardening tools, or sports equipment.
- **Projects:** Begin a new project that you are passionate about, whether it be a craft, home renovation, or learning a new skill.
- **Memberships:** Consider joining or subscribing to a streaming service, magazine, or group that interests you.

4. Social Activities:

- **Outings with Friends:** Organize a fun outing with friends, such as a picnic, game night, or hiking trip.
- **Family Time:** Spend meaningful time with your family doing activities that everyone enjoys, such as a BBQ, beach day, or board game night.
- **Support Groups:** Participate in support group activities that celebrate accomplishments together.

5. Personal Treats:

- **Shopping:** Indulge in new experiences, such as shopping for clothing, books, or gadgets.
- **Pampering:** Enjoy pampering treatments such as a manicure, pedicure, or haircut.
- **Home Comforts:** Purchase items to make your living place more comfortable or delightful, such as a soft blanket, scented candles, or plants.

How to Implement a Rewards System

1. Define Your Goals:

- **Clear goals:** Clearly outline your short- and long-term goals. Make sure your goals are specific, measurable, achievable, relevant, and time-bound (SMART).
- **Milestones:** Divide major goals into smaller milestones that are easier to accomplish and track.

2. Match Rewards with Goals:

- **Appropriate rewards:** Adjust the size of the award to reflect the difficulty and relevance of the goal. Fewer goals can have fewer rewards, whereas larger successes can offer more substantial benefits.
- **List of rewards:** Make a list of potential prizes and match them to specific goals or achievements.

3. Track your progress:

- **Progress Log:** Keep track of your progress towards each target. This can be done in a journal, planner, or through a digital tool.
- **Celebrate Success:** When you achieve a goal, take the time to completely enjoy your prize.

4. Be flexible:

- **Adjust as needed:** Be willing to change your reward scheme as needed. If specific rewards aren't motivating you, try something different.
- **Reflect:** Check in on what rewards are working effectively and make improvements to keep the system successful and pleasant.

Maintaining Motivation Throughout the Recovery Journey

Maintaining motivation during your ARFID recovery journey might be difficult, but it is necessary for long-term development.

Understanding Motivation During Recovery

Motivation is the driving factor behind setting and achieving goals. Maintaining motivation in the context of ARFID rehabilitation requires both internal elements (such as personal desires and values) and external factors (such as social support and environmental influences).

Strategies to Maintain Motivation

1. Set Clear and Achievable Goals:

- **SMART Goals:** Set specific, measurable, attainable, relevant, and time-bound (SMART) goals. Clear goals provide direction and make it easy to monitor progress.
- **Break down goals:** Break down larger ambitions into smaller, more achievable actions. This makes the rehabilitation process less overwhelming and allows for more consistent progress.

2. Celebrate Small Victories:

- **Acknowledge Progress:** Recognize and celebrate every minor win along the way. Every step forward is noteworthy and should be recognized.
- **Reward Yourself:** Use a reward system to reinforce good behavior. Choose rewards that are meaningful and fun for you.

3. Keep a Recovery Journal:

- **Follow Your Journey:** Keep a journal to record your ideas, feelings, and progress. Writing about your experiences allows you to reflect on your path while remaining focused on your goals.
- **Find Patterns:** Journaling can help you find patterns and triggers, revealing areas that need to be addressed and improved.

4. Create a Strong Support System

- **Engage family and friends:** Surround yourself with supportive relatives and friends who understand your challenges and celebrate your accomplishments.
- **Join Supporting Groups:** Join a support group, either in person or online, to connect with others going through similar circumstances. Sharing and hearing other people's tales can be quite encouraging.

5. Focus on the Positive:

- **Positive Self-Talk:** Use positive self-talk to overcome negative ideas and improve confidence. Remind yourself of your strengths and accomplishments.
- **Appreciation:** Develop a sense of appreciation by consistently noticing the good things in your life and recovery process.

6. Visualise Success:

- **Imagery Techniques:** Use imagery tools to see your success and the benefits of your work. This mental activity might help you gain motivation and confidence.
- **Vision Boards:** Make a vision board with images and statements that reflect your aims and desires. Place it somewhere you'll see it every day to remind yourself of your goals.

7. Be flexible and adaptable:

- **Adjust goals:** Be open to changing your goals and techniques as necessary. Flexibility guarantees that failures do not derail your development and that you can adapt to new conditions.
- **Learn from Setbacks:** View setbacks as learning experiences rather than failures. Think about what went wrong and how you might do better going forward.

8. Prioritise Self-Care:

- **Physical Health:** Maintain physical health by obtaining enough sleep, eating good meals, and exercising regularly. Physical well-being promotes mental and emotional resiliency.
- **Mental Health:** Take part in activities that enhance mental well-being, such as mindfulness practices, relaxation techniques, and hobbies you enjoy.

9. Seek Professional Support:

- **Therapists and Counselors:** Seek professional support from therapists and counselors. Consult with a therapist or counselor who specializes in ARFID and eating disorders. Professional advice can provide useful tools and ideas for staying motivated.
- **Medical support:** Regular check-ins with your healthcare practitioner guarantee that your physical health is properly monitored and controlled.

10. Remind Yourself of Why:

- **Personal Reasons:** Regularly remind yourself of why you started your recovery path. Whether you want to better your health, enjoy social activities, or attain personal goals, remembering your "why" helps you stay motivated.
- **Visual reminders:** Use visual reminders, such as notes, images, or items, to represent your motivations for recovery. Place them in prominent

locations to maintain your motivation.

IV

Part 4: Finding Your Voice: Sharing Your ARFID Story

8

Chapter 8: The Power of Sharing Your ARFID Story

Why Sharing Your Story Matters

Raising awareness of Avoidant Restrictive Food Intake Disorder (ARFID) and refuting prevalent misunderstandings is critical for increasing understanding and support for individuals affected. By educating the public and dispelling myths, we can foster a more caring and informed community.

Importance of Raising Awareness

Awareness is the first step towards acceptance and assistance. When others understand ARFID and how it impacts people, they are more inclined to provide compassion and aid. Raising awareness helps:

- **Reduce stigma:** Educating others about ARFID can assist in decreasing the stigma and shame associated with the illness, encouraging those who are affected to seek treatment.
- **Promote early intervention:** Increased awareness allows for earlier

detection and intervention, greatly improving outcomes for people with ARFID.

- **Encourage Research and Resources:** Raising awareness can lead to more funding for research and resource development, resulting in improved treatment options and support networks.

Myths and Facts About ARFID

Myth 1: ARFID is simply picky eating.

- **Fact:** ARFID is more than just finicky eating. While picky eaters may have preferences and dislikes, people with ARFID have extreme food avoidance, which can result in nutritional deficits, weight loss, and impairments in everyday functioning. Sensory sensitivities, fear of choking, or a lack of interest in eating are common reasons for avoidance, and they are far more acute and limiting than usual picky eating behaviors.

Myth 2: People with ARFID Don't Want to Eat.

- **Fact:** In reality, they may experience anxiety, sensory difficulties, or bodily reactions that make eating challenging. They may want to eat more or try new foods, but their condition makes this difficult.

Myth 3: There is a "cure" for ARFID.

- **Fact:** There is no one-size-fits-all treatment for ARFID. Treatment frequently includes a combination of therapies customized to the individual's needs, such as cognitive-behavioral therapy (CBT), exposure therapy, and dietary counseling. Managing ARFID entails devising techniques to cope with and eventually overcome food aversions and anxieties.

Myth 4: ARFID is a phase that children outgrow.

- **Fact:** While some children outgrow fussy eating habits, ARFID is a significant eating condition that can last into adulthood if not treated properly. Early intervention is critical for avoiding long-term health repercussions and promoting healthier eating habits.

Myth 5: ARFID only affects children.

- **Fact:** While ARFID is commonly found in youngsters, it can affect people of any age. Many individuals deal with ARFID, and the disorder can affect anyone, regardless of age, gender, or background.

Myth 6: ARFID is a result of bad parenting.

- **Fact:** ARFID is not caused by parenting styles or behaviors. It is a multifaceted illness having genetic, psychological, and environmental components. Blaming parents is not only incorrect but also detrimental and counterproductive.

Strategies For Raising Awareness

1. Education and Advocacy:

- **Share information:** Use social media, blogs, and public speaking opportunities to spread factual information about ARFID. Emphasise personal stories and experiences to humanize the condition and develop empathy.
- **Hosting Workshops & Seminars:** Organise educational workshops and seminars for schools, healthcare providers, and community organizations to promote ARFID understanding and awareness.
- **Collaborate with Advocacy Groups:** To amplify your efforts and reach a larger audience, work with eating disorder advocacy groups and organizations.

2. Media and Publicity:

- **Press releases and articles:** Write press releases and articles for local newspapers, journals, and websites to raise awareness about ARFID.
- **Interviews and Features:** Share ARFID-related information and personal experiences through interviews and feature stories on radio, television, and podcasts.
- **Public Service Announcements:** Create and disseminate public service messages (PSAs) regarding ARFID to raise awareness and support for individuals affected.

3. Community Involvement:

- **Support Groups:** Create or promote support groups for people with ARFID and their families. These groups offer a secure environment in which to share experiences, receive support, and learn from one another.
- **School Programmes:** Collaborate with schools to establish programs that educate students, teachers, and parents about ARFID and other eating disorders. This may include classroom presentations, instructional leaflets, and staff training sessions.
- **Health Fairs and Events:** Attend health fairs and community events to distribute educational materials and engage the public in conversations regarding ARFID.

4. Online Resources:

- **Educational Websites:** Create or contribute to educational websites with detailed information about ARFID, including symptoms, treatment options, and support services.
- **Social Media Campaigns:** Use hashtags, infographics, and personal stories to raise awareness and dispel misinformation about ARFID. Encourage followers to share the information with a larger audience.
- **Online Support Communities:** Create online support groups where people

with ARFID and their families may connect, share stories, and find resources.

Connecting with Others Who Understand

Finding connection and understanding is critical for those afflicted with ARFID. Engaging with others who have had similar situations can offer emotional support, practical assistance, and a feeling of community.

Advantages of Connecting with Others

1. Emotional Support:

- **Shared Experiences:** Sharing experiences can provide consolation in knowing you are not alone in your problems. Sharing experiences with people who understand ARFID promotes empathy and validation.
- **Encouragement and Hope:** Hearing about other people's accomplishments and problems gives you encouragement and hope, which motivates you to continue your recovery journey.

2. Practical Advice:

- **Coping practices:** Experienced individuals with ARFID can share their successful coping practices.
- **Resource Sharing:** Communities frequently share vital resources including therapists, nutritionists, support groups, and instructional materials.

3. Building Community:

- **Sense of Belonging:** Connecting with others who understand ARFID promotes a sense of belonging and reduces feelings of isolation and loneliness.

- **Mutual Support:** In a supportive community, individuals may rely on one another for assistance, forming a network of mutual support and understanding.

Ways to Connect

1. Online Support Communities and Forums:

- **Social Media Groups:** Social media platforms such as Facebook and Reddit offer ARFID-specific communities for members to share stories, ask questions, and offer support.
- **Specialized Forums:** Websites like ARFID Awareness UK and other eating disorder help sites frequently feature ARFID-specific forums.

2. In-Person Support Groups:

- **Local groups:** Look for local support groups in hospitals, clinics, or community centers that meet for people with ARFID and their families.
- **Therapy Groups:** Some therapists provide group therapy sessions for people suffering from eating disorders, such as ARFID. These can create an organized setting for sharing and support.

3. ARFID Advocacy Groups and Resources:

- **Nonprofit Organisations:** The National Eating Disorders Association (NEDA) and ARFID Awareness UK provide materials, support networks, and events related to ARFID.
- **Workshops and Conferences:** Attending workshops and conferences on eating disorders allows you to meet others who understand ARFID and learn from specialists.

4. Social Media and Blogs:

- **Blogging:** Create or follow ARFID blogs to share your story and connect with others who are on the same journey. Blogs can be an effective tool for sharing experiences and building community.
- **Instagram and Twitter:** Use hashtags such as #ARFID, #ARFIDRecovery, and #EatingDisorders to identify and interact with others on these sites.

5. Professional Networks:

- **Therapists and Dietitians:** Ask your therapist or dietician about support groups or networks for individuals with ARFID.
- **Healthcare Providers:** Some healthcare providers offer support programs or can connect you with local or online networks.

Tips for Developing Connections

1. Be open and honest.

- **Share your story:** Open up about your experiences with ARFID. Honesty can assist in fostering trust and improve relationships with people.
- **Active Listening:** When others share their stories, pay close attention. Empathy and understanding promote a helpful environment.

2. Participate Regularly:

- **Consistent Engagement:** Regular engagement in support groups or online forums fosters relationships and provides continuing support.
- **Contribute Positively:** Share positive thoughts and encouragement with others to foster a helpful and inspiring environment.

3. Seek Diverse Perspectives:

- **Variety of Experiences:** Engage with individuals from diverse backgrounds and experiences to gain different perspectives and coping strategies.

- **Inclusive Community:** Encourage an inclusive environment where everyone feels welcome and valued.

4. Respect Boundaries:

- **Personal Comfort Levels:** Respect the boundaries and comfort levels of others in the community. Not everyone may be ready to share their experiences in detail.
- **Confidentiality:** Maintain confidentiality and respect the privacy of others, fostering a safe and trusting environment.

5. Use Available Resources:

- **Educational resources:** Share and apply educational resources supplied by support groups and organizations to improve comprehension and coping skills.
- **Professional Help:** Encourage getting professional help when needed, emphasizing that support groups are a supplement to, not a replacement for, professional therapy.

Finding Inspiration and Hope Through Shared Experiences

Navigating the issues of ARFID can be stressful and alienating. However, connecting with others who have had similar experiences can be a source of hope and inspiration. Shared experiences provide helpful insights, encouragement, and a reminder that you are not alone on your journey.

The Power of Shared Experiences

1. Validation and Understanding:

- **Feel understood:** Hearing from others who have gone through similar problems can bring a powerful sense of validation. Knowing that others understand what you're going through can be comforting.
- **Shared Emotions:** Having comparable sensations of anxiety, dread, and irritation can lead to a strong emotional connection and mutual understanding.

2. Learning and Growth:

- **Practical Tips:** Stories of how others have dealt with ARFID can provide practical ideas and coping processes that you may not have considered.
- **Encouragement to explore New Things:** Witnessing others' success in their recovery journeys might motivate you to explore new ways and push yourself beyond your comfort zone.

3. Fostering Hope and Resilience:

- **Success Stories:** Hearing success stories from others who have made substantial progress in managing ARFID might inspire and motivate you to continue your efforts.
- **Strength in Numbers:** Knowing that others have experienced and overcome similar struggles helps boost your resilience and motivation to keep going.

How to Find and Share Experiences

1. Supporting Groups:

- **In-Person Meetings:** Join local support groups to meet people in person, share stories, and provide mutual support. Such gatherings are frequently held in hospitals, clinics, and community centers.
- **Online communities:** Participate in ARFID-related forums and social media communities. These platforms allow you to share your stories, ask questions, and provide support from the comfort of your own home.

2. Personal Blogs and Vlogs:

- **Writing Blogs:** Create or follow blogs where individuals share their experiences with ARFID. Writing your blog might help you digest your experiences and connect with others.
- **Video Journals:** Watch or produce vlogs about your personal experiences with ARFID. Seeing and hearing from people can foster a stronger personal connection.

3. Advocacy and Awareness Events:

- **Workshops and Seminars:** Attend eating disorder-related events to hear from specialists and others who have shared their experiences.
- **Conferences:** Attend conferences that bring together people with ARFID, their families, and healthcare experts to share information and experiences.

4. Social Media Platforms:

- **Hashtags and Groups:** Use hashtags like #ARFIDJourney, #ARFIDRecovery, and #EatingDisorders to identify and connect with others on social media platforms such as Instagram, Twitter, and Facebook.

- **Sharing Your Story:** If you feel comfortable, share your own experiences on social media. This can motivate others and generate a chain reaction of support and understanding.

5. Books and Articles:

- **Personal Accounts:** Read books and articles that share personal experiences with ARFID. These stories might offer perspective and motivation.
- **Writing Your Story:** Consider writing about your personal experiences for blogs, articles, or novels. Your story can be an effective tool for raising awareness and providing hope to others.

Finding Your Voice: Connecting with Others Who Understand

Connecting with others who understand ARFID's unique challenges can provide invaluable support, encouragement, and a feeling of community. Online support groups and forums offer a handy and accessible method to share stories, seek advice, and feel better knowing you're not alone.

Benefits of Online Support Groups and Forums.

1. Accessibility and Convenience:

- **24/7 Access:** Online support groups are open around the clock, allowing you to seek help and share your experiences whenever necessary.
- **Global Community:** Connect with individuals from all over the world to acquire new insights and support from a large community.

2. Anonymity and Privacy:

- **Confidentiality:** Many online forums allow users to post anonymously, making it simpler to discuss personal stories and seek assistance without fear of being judged.
- **Safe Space:** Online communities frequently offer a safe and non-judgmental atmosphere in which to openly discuss your issues and progress.

3. Peer Support:

- **Shared Experiences:** Connecting with people who share similar situations can offer emotional support and practical counsel from firsthand knowledge.
- **Encouragement:** Online groups provide a forum for both giving and receiving support, which can help you stay motivated throughout your recovery journey.

Recommended Online Support Groups and Forums

1. Facebook Groups:

- **ARFID Support Groups:** Look for ARFID-specific groups on Facebook, like "ARFID Support Group" or "ARFID Parents Support Group." These communities frequently have thousands of members and engage in active conversations.
- **Eating Disorder Communities:** Broader eating disorder support groups, such as the "Eating Disorder Support Network," might be beneficial because they frequently include people with ARFID.

2. Reddit communities:

- **r/ARFID:** This subreddit is for people with ARFID and provides a forum for sharing experiences, asking questions, and offering mutual support.

- **r/EatingDisorders:** A bigger subreddit for eating disorders, including postings and debates around ARFID.

3. Specialised Forums:

- **ARFID Awareness UK :** Provides forums for persons with ARFID to share stories, seek assistance, and access resources.
- **Beat Eating Disorders:** Beat, the UK's premier eating disorder charity, provides online support groups and forums, including those for ARFID.

4. Eating Disorder Websites:

- **National Eating Disorders Association (NEDA):** The National Eating Disorders Association (NEDA) provides forums and online chat groups to interact with others experiencing similar issues.
- **Something Fishy:** Something Fishy is an online resource dedicated to eating disorder recovery. It offers forums and chat rooms for support and education.

5. Social Media Platforms:

- **Instagram:** On Instagram, use hashtags such as #ARFID, #ARFIDRecovery, and #EatingDisorders to connect with others sharing their experiences.
- **Twitter:** Follow and interact with accounts dedicated to ARFID and eating disorder awareness to participate in conversations and get support.

ARFID Advocacy Organizations and Resources

Advocacy organizations and websites dedicated to ARFID serve an important role in raising awareness, offering support, and providing essential information to individuals and families impacted by this eating disease. These organizations frequently offer educational resources, support networks, and opportunities for lobbying and policy change.

Leading advocacy organizations

1. Visit the National Eating Disorders Association (NEDA)

- **Website:** NEDA
- **Overview:** The National Eating Disorders Association is one of the largest organizations dedicated to eating disorders in the United States. They provide materials, support groups, and advocacy campaigns geared specifically towards ARFID and other eating disorders.
- **Resources:** NEDA offers instructional materials, hotlines, and opportunities to connect with others through support groups and events.

2. ARFID Awareness UK

- **Website:** ARFID Awareness UK
- **Overview:** This organization works to raise awareness of ARFID in the United Kingdom. They offer information to individuals, families, and healthcare professionals.
- **Resources:** ARFID Awareness UK provides online forums, informational articles, and a venue for sharing personal stories to assist raise awareness and understanding of ARFID.

3. Beat Eating Disorders

- **Website:** Beat Eating Disorders
- **Overview:** Beat is a leading UK-based organization that helps people with eating disorders, including ARFID. They provide a variety of services, including helplines, support groups, and instructional resources.
- **Resources:** Beat offers online support groups, helplines, professional training, and awareness campaigns to help people with ARFID understand

and support themselves.

4. F.E.A.S.T. (Families Empowered and Supporting Treatment of Eating Disorders)

- **Website:** F.E.A.S.T.
- **Overview:** An international organization that assists families afflicted by eating disorders. They offer tools and advocacy specifically for carers and relatives of people with ARFID and other eating disorders.
- **Resources:** F.E.A.S.T. provides instructional resources, online forums, and a platform for families to share their experiences and support one another.

Key Resources and Tools

1. Educational resources and guides

- **NEDA Toolkit:** NEDA provides toolkits for parents, educators, and healthcare professionals that contain information on identifying and managing ARFID.
- **Beat's Resources:** Beat offers extensive guidelines and factsheets on ARFID, including symptoms, treatment choices, and how to help a loved one.

2. Helplines & Hotlines

- **NEDA Helpline:** NEDA provides a discreet helpline for people looking for information and support. You can contact them at 1-800-931-2237.
- **Beat Helpline:** For those in the UK, call 0808 801 0677. They also provide email and web chat help.

3. Online support groups and forums.

- **NEDA Online Groups:** NEDA provides virtual support groups in which people can interact with others who are facing similar issues.
- **ARFID Awareness UK Forums:** This platform allows persons with ARFID to share their stories, ask questions, and seek help.

4. Advocacy and Awareness Campaigns

- **Eating disorders:** Many organizations, including NEDA and Beat, have annual awareness weeks to increase understanding and support for eating disorders.
- **ARFID-Specific Campaigns:** Organisations such as ARFID Awareness UK conduct targeted campaigns to promote awareness and fight for better treatment and support for those living with ARFID.

5. Professional Training and Development

- **Beat Training:** Beat provides training programs for healthcare professionals to increase their knowledge and treatment of ARFID.
- **NEDA seminars:** NEDA offers seminars and webinars for professionals and carers to help them improve their knowledge and abilities in assisting people with ARFID.

Sharing Your Story on Social Media Platforms (if comfortable)

Sharing your ARFID experience on social media can be an effective method to promote awareness, connect with others, and seek help. While it might be difficult to open up about personal problems, the benefits of telling your experience generally exceed the risks, as long as you feel comfortable and safe doing so.

Benefits of Sharing Your Story

1. Raising Awareness:

- **Educational Impact:** Sharing personal experiences can help others understand ARFID and dispel misinformation about the illness.
- **Broad Reach:** Social media enables you to reach a large audience, providing awareness and information to people who may not be familiar with ARFID.

2. Finding Support:

- **Community Building:** Building a community with individuals who share similar experiences helps foster a sense of belonging and support.
- **Empathy and Encouragement:** Sharing your story may elicit empathetic responses and encouragement from others, increasing your morale and resilience.

3. Empowerment:

- **Owning Your Narrative:** Telling your story in your own words can boost confidence and give you control over your journey.
- **Inspiration:** Your story can inspire others who are struggling, giving them hope and determination to get assistance and continue their recovery.

Tips for Sharing Your Story

1. Select the Right Platform:

- **Instagram:** Instagram is ideal for sharing visual content like images, graphics, and videos. Use hashtags such as #ARFID, #ARFIDAwareness, and #EatingDisorderRecovery to reach a targeted audience.

- **Facebook:** Facebook is ideal for longer posts and interacting with support groups. Join ARFID-specific organizations to reach a certain audience.
- **Twitter:** Twitter is an excellent platform for short updates and conversations. Follow and use hashtags to participate in bigger conversations around eating disorders and mental health.
- **YouTube:** YouTube is ideal for sharing in-depth video material. Create vlogs to capture your journey and provide insights regarding life with ARFID.

2. Prioritise your comfort and safety:

- **Anonymity:** If you want to stay anonymous, choose a pseudonym or tell your experience without disclosing personal information.
- **Privacy Settings:** Change your privacy settings to limit who may view your posts. Consider sharing with a small group of friends or followers first.
- **Boundaries:** Determine what portions of your tale you are willing to share. You don't have to disclose everything; just focus on what you believe is relevant and manageable.

3. Be Honest and Authentic:

- **Real Experiences:** Share your actual experiences, both obstacles and successes. Authenticity connects with others and builds stronger relationships.
- **Emotional Honesty:** It is acceptable to communicate vulnerabilities and feelings. Sharing your feelings might help others empathize with your situation and provide real assistance.

4. Use Visuals and Multimedia:

- **Photos and Videos:** Adding photos and videos to your tale can increase engagement. Share photographs, infographics, or films that depict your experience and insights.

- **Creative Expression:** Express yourself creatively through narrative, poetry, or art. Creativity may improve your message and increase its effect.

5. Engage Your Audience:

- **Respond to comments:** Engage with those who leave comments on your posts. Answering questions and providing feedback might help to build a helpful discourse.
- **Join Conversations:** Participate in debates and exchange useful stuff from others. Engaging with the community can help you grow your support network and spread your message.

Potential Challenges and How to Address them

1. Negative Feedback:

- **Stay Positive:** When receiving negative feedback, be optimistic and focus on encouraging responses. Remember that nasty remarks are typically about the commenter rather than you.
- **Moderate Comments:** Use moderation tools to remove harmful or inappropriate comments. Block or report users who exhibit abusive behavior.

2. Emotional Impact:

- **Self-Care:** Prioritize your mental wellness. If you're feeling overwhelmed, take a vacation from social media and do something for yourself.
- **Seek Help:** If sharing your story triggers strong emotions, contact trustworthy friends, family, or mental health specialists.

3. Privacy concerns:

- **Control Information:** Be wary of the personal information you disclose. Avoid providing information that may jeopardize your privacy or safety.
- **Selective Sharing:** If you're concerned about your story's public visibility, consider sharing it in closed or private groups instead.

Building a Community: Resources and Support Groups for ARFID

Connecting with people who are experiencing ARFID can be beneficial. This shared experience generates a sense of camaraderie, understanding, and mutual support, which can significantly improve your recovery process. Here are some significant benefits of interacting with others facing similar issues.

Emotional Support

1. Feeling Understood:

- **Shared Experiences:** Interacting with those who have ARFID means connecting with people who understand your difficulties. This shared understanding can bring consolation and alleviate feelings of loneliness.
- **Empathy:** People with comparable experiences can provide empathy and affirmation, which can be quite soothing in stressful times.

2. Reducing Isolation:

- **Building Friendships:** Developing Friendships Connecting with individuals who have ARFID can lead to meaningful friendships, alleviating feelings of loneliness and isolation.
- **Support Networks:** Being a part of a supportive community can give you with a consistent network of people to turn to for encouragement and

advice.

Practical advice

1. Learning from Others:

- **Shared Strategies:** Sharing coping strategies, suggestions, and tactics from others with ARFID might provide valuable insights that may not be available elsewhere.
- **Problem-Solving:** Discussing problems with peers can lead to new answers and techniques for managing symptoms, making daily living easier.

2. Navigating Treatment:

- **Therapy Recommendations:** Connecting with others might help you find effective therapists, dietitians, and treatment programs for ARFID.
- **Resource Sharing:** Peers can recommend useful resources such as books, websites, and support groups to help you expand your knowledge and network.

Inspiration & Motivation

1. Observing Progress:

- **Role Models:** Watching others make success in their recovery can be motivational and motivating, demonstrating that improvement is achievable.
- **Success Stories:** Hearing about others' accomplishments, no matter how minor, can give you hope and support for your journey.

2. Accountability:

- **Goal Setting:** Setting goals with others helps increase commitment to recovery.
- **Mutual encouragement:** Encouraging one another to stick to treatment goals and attempt new tactics can increase motivation and perseverance.

Shared Resources

1. Access to Information:

- **Educational Materials:** Connecting with others can provide essential educational materials to further your understanding of ARFID.
- **Seminars and Webinars:** Peers may provide information on forthcoming events, seminars, or webinars that will help you on your recovery journey.

2. Collaborative Learning:

- **Group Discussions:** Group conversations provide opportunities for varied viewpoints and ideas, increasing knowledge and coping skills.
- **Resource Pools:** Being a member of a community gives you access to a common pool of resources and knowledge that is often more comprehensive than what you could find on your own.

Advocacy & Awareness

1. Collective Voice:

- **Raising Awareness:** By joining forces with others, you can participate in advocacy efforts to raise awareness about ARFID, contributing to a broader understanding and acceptance of the disorder.
- **Policy Change:** Working with others can help you advocate for greater treatment alternatives, insurance coverage, and research funding.

2. Community Projects:

- **Support Initiatives:** Participate in support initiatives, such as building support groups, organizing events, or developing educational campaigns, by connecting with others.
- **Volunteering:** Working with ARFID-focused organizations alongside peers can give you a feeling of purpose while also benefiting the community.

Finding Local Support Groups or Therapy Groups Focused on ARFID

Finding local support groups or therapy groups that specialize in ARFID can be a crucial part of your recovery path. These groups offer a secure environment in which to share experiences, acquire insights, and receive support from others who understand what you're going through. Here are some methods and suggestions to help you find these resources:

1. Start with online searches.

1. Use specific keywords.

- **Search terms:** Search for "ARFID support groups near me," "ARFID therapy groups in [your city]," or "eating disorder support groups focused on ARFID."
- **Location-Based Search:** Include your city or region in the search to limit the results to local options.

2. Check specialized websites:

- **Eating Disorder Organisations:** The websites of organizations such as the National Eating Disorders Association (NEDA), Eating Disorders

Anonymous (EDA), and local eating disorder advocacy groups frequently include support group directories.

- **Hospital and Clinic Websites:** Many hospitals and clinics that specialize in eating disorders have websites with information about their support groups and therapy alternatives.

2. Reach out to healthcare providers.

1. Consult your therapist or doctor:

- **Referrals:** Your present therapist, doctor, or nutritionist may be aware of local support or therapy groups focusing on ARFID.
- **Professional Networks:** Healthcare providers frequently have professional networks and can connect you to credible group leaders and programs.

2. Contact the Eating Disorder Clinic:

- **Local clinics:** Contact your local eating disorder clinics. They may offer group therapy sessions tailored to ARFID or provide information on neighboring support groups.
- **Specialized Programmes:** Some clinics provide intensive outpatient (IOP) or partial hospitalization (PHP) programs with group treatment components.

3. Use Community Resources.

1. Libraries and Community Centers:

- **Bulletin Boards:** Check bulletin boards at local libraries, community centers, and wellness centers for information about support groups.

- **Community Programmes:** Some community centers provide mental health support services, including those for eating disorders.

2. Colleges and Universities:

- **Campus Health Services:** If you are a student, please contact the campus health or counseling services. They may provide support groups or link you to local services.
- **Psychology Departments:** Universities with psychology or counseling programs may offer support groups as part of their training clinics.

4. Consider Online and Hybrid Options.

1. Online Directories:

- **Eating Disorder Support Networks**: Websites like NEDA, EDA, and the Alliance for Eating Disorders Awareness frequently feature both in-person and online support groups.
- **Therapist Directories:** Platforms like Psychology Today allow you to search for therapists and group treatment alternatives based on region and specialty, including ARFID.

2. Hybrid Groups:

- **Combination Meetings:** Some groups combine in-person and online meetings for greater flexibility and accessibility. This is especially useful if you can't find a local group or want to take a hybrid approach.

5. Participate in social media and online communities.

1. Social Media Groups:

- **Facebook Groups:** Look for ARFID-specific support groups on Facebook. Some of these groups may have members in your region who may recommend in-person activities.
- **Instagram and Reddit:** Follow ARFID-related hashtags on Instagram or join relevant subreddits to interact with others and discover local resources.

2. Online Forums:

- **Eating Disorder Forums:** Websites such as Beat Eating Disorders and Eating Disorder Hope offer forums for participants to share resources, including local support groups.
- **Parent and Carer Networks:** If you are a parent or carer, check for forums and groups dedicated to supporting individuals with ARFID. They frequently share helpful resources and recommendations.

6. Attend related events and workshops.

1. Conferences and Workshops:

- **Eating Disorder Conferences:** Attend eating disorder-related conferences, courses, or seminars. These gatherings frequently have networking opportunities, allowing you to meet experts and peers who can recommend local support organizations.
- **Community Events:** Participate in community events that promote mental health and wellness. These events may feature information booths or presentations about eating disorder support resources.

2. Health Fairs and Expos:

- **Local Health Events:** Attend health fairs and expos near you. Organizations and clinics that take part in these events frequently provide information about their services, including support groups.

The Importance of Building a Network of Support

Building a support network is critical for people suffering from Avoidant/Restrictive Food Intake Disorder (ARFID). This support network, which includes family, friends, healthcare professionals, and peers, can provide vital emotional, practical, and motivational support. Here are the main reasons why creating a robust support network is vital for controlling ARFID:

Emotional Support

1. Validation and Understanding:

- **Shared Experiences:** Connecting with others who use ARFID provides a sense of validation. Knowing that others understand your challenges helps to alleviate feelings of isolation.
- **Empathy:** Supportive people show empathy and compassion, making it easier to deal with the emotional difficulties connected with ARFID.

2. Reducing Isolation:

- **Combatting Loneliness:** Creating a support network can alleviate loneliness associated with ARFID, providing a sense of belonging and camaraderie.
- **Peer Encouragement:** Interacting with people who have had similar experiences can provide encouragement and hope, leading to a more optimistic attitude toward recovery.

Practical Assistance

1. Access to Resources:

- **Resource Sharing:** Your network can provide helpful information about therapy alternatives, therapists, and dietitians who specialize in ARFID.
- **Practical Tips:** Peers can offer practical advice on symptom management, such as ideas for broadening your food options or dealing with sensory aversions.

2. Collaborative Problem-Solving:

- **Group Discussions:** Group talks facilitate brainstorming and problem-solving, bringing varied viewpoints and ideas.
- **Learning from Others:** Hearing about others' accomplishments and problems can offer you ideas and solutions to use on your journey.

Enhancing Treatment and Recovery

1. Encouragement and motivation:

- **Setting Goals:** Supportive people can help you set realistic goals and celebrate your successes, increasing your motivation to continue with treatment.
- **Accountability:** Knowing that others are interested in your development fosters a sense of accountability, which encourages commitment to treatment regimens.

2. Professional Referrals:

- **Recommendations:** Ask your support network, including healthcare providers, for recommendations on ARFID-focused experts or groups.

- **Navigating the system:** Others' advice can help you navigate the health-care system more successfully and ensure you receive thorough care.

Building Resilience.

1. Emotional Resilience:

- **Coping Mechanisms:** Learning from others' coping techniques can assist manage anxiety, despair, and stress associated with ARFID.
- **Self-Compassion:** Encouragement from your network promotes self-compassion and acceptance, which are essential for overcoming negative self-perceptions.

2. Support During Challenges:

- **Crisis Management:** Having a strong network can provide quick assistance and understanding during setbacks or difficult times.
- **Long-Term Stability:** A solid support network offers continuous stability and reassurance while you navigate the ups and downs of recovery.

Advocacy & Awareness

1. Amplifying Voices:

- **Advocacy Efforts:** Work together to raise awareness and understanding of ARFID among healthcare practitioners and the community.
- **Sharing Stories:** Sharing personal experiences among your network will help dispel myths and educate people about the realities of living with ARFID.

V

Part 5: A Look to the Future: Living a Fulfilling Life with ARFID

9

Chapter 9: Living Well with ARFID: Strategies for Long-Term Management

Maintaining a Healthy Relationship with Food

Intuitive eating promotes a healthy relationship with food by increasing awareness of the body's natural hunger and satiety cues. Individuals with ARFID may benefit most from practicing intuitive eating practices since they assist in rebuilding confidence in their bodies and foster a more positive, balanced connection with food.

Understanding Intuitive Eating

1. Listen to Your Body:

- **Hunger and Fullness Cues:** Intuitive eating focuses on understanding your body's hunger and fullness signals. Learning to recognize and respond to these signs can help you eat in a way that is appropriate for your body.
- **Mindful Eating:** Practice being present throughout meals, focusing on the flavor, texture, and contentment that comes from eating. This can

help you become more aware of your body's responses to various foods.

2. Rejecting Diet Mentality:

- **Avoiding Food Rules:** Intuitive eating supports breaking free from restrictive diets and food regulations, which can lead to feelings of guilt or worry over eating. Instead, concentrate on fueling your body and eating without judgment.
- **Embracing All Foods:** Allow yourself to consume a range of foods without categorizing them as "good" or "bad." This reduces the dread and anxiety associated with eating.

Practical Steps to Intuitive Eating

1. Start Slowly and steadily:

- **Small changes:** Begin with minor, attainable modifications to your dietary habits. Introduce new foods gradually and pay attention to your body's responses.
- **Patience:** Developing intuitive eating habits takes time, particularly for those with ARFID. Be patient with yourself, and understand that development may be sluggish.

2. Keep a Food Journal:

- **Tracking Hunger and Fullness:** Keep a food journal to track what you eat and how you feel before, during, and after meals. Track your hunger and fullness levels to find patterns and areas for improvement.
- **Emotional Connections:** Focus on the emotional components of eating. Understanding how emotions affect your eating patterns might help you create healthier coping strategies.

3. Create a Positive Eating Environment:

- **Setting the Scene:** Make your dining area a relaxing and comfortable place. To truly engage in the eating experience, avoid distractions such as television and phones.
- **Enjoying Meals:** Make mealtimes more fun by including your favorite meals and experimenting with new dishes. This can assist in relieving anxiety and make eating more enjoyable.

Overcoming Challenges

1. Addressing Fear Foods:

- **Gradual Exposure:** Reintroduce fear foods into your diet in a controlled, supportive atmosphere. Reduce anxiety by pairing these items with safe, familiar options.
- **Positive Reinforcement:** Recognise little triumphs when trying new meals. Positive reinforcement can help to increase confidence and lessen fear over time.

2. Managing Sensory Issues:

- **Sensory-Friendly Foods:** Choose foods that match your sensory preferences (e.g. texture, fragrance, appearance) and progressively broaden your diet.
- **Desensitization procedures:** Collaborate with a therapist or nutritionist to develop desensitization procedures that can help lessen sensory aversions and expand food options.

3. Seeking Professional Support:

- **Therapist Guidance:** A therapist who specializes in eating disorders can help you address the psychological aspects of ARFID and support your journey to intuitive eating.

- **Dietitian Assistance:** A trained dietitian can provide personalized nutrition advice and assist you in creating a balanced, intuitive eating plan that is tailored to your specific needs.

Benefits of Intuitive Eating

1. Improved Relationship with Food:

- **Reduced Anxiety:** Intuitive eating alleviates food-related anxiety by eliminating the need to follow rigorous diets and guidelines.
- **Increased Enjoyment:** Concentrating on the pleasure of eating can result in a more pleasant and fulfilling connection with food.

2. Improved Physical Health:

- **Balanced Nutrition:** Intuitive eating encourages a balanced, varied diet that fits your body's nutritional requirements, thereby boosting general health and well-being.
- **Sustainable Habits:** Unlike restrictive diets, intuitive eating promotes long-term eating habits that are easier to stick to.

3. Improved Emotional Well-Being:

- **Body Trust:** Rebuilding faith in your body's cues for hunger and fullness can boost self-esteem and body image.
- **Emotional Resilience:** Practicing intuitive eating can boost emotional resilience, allowing you to manage better with stress and emotional issues.

Focusing on Nourishment and Enjoyment

When dealing with ARFID (Avoidant/Restrictive Eating Intake Disorder), it is critical to change the emphasis towards sustenance and enjoyment of eating. This strategy not only meets nutritional demands but also promotes a healthier, more positive connection with food. Here are some basic ideas to help you focus on both nourishing your body and enjoying the dining experience:

Prioritizing Nourishment

1. Balanced Nutrition:

- **Nutrient-Dense Foods:** Aim to eat a variety of nutrient-dense foods. These foods include necessary vitamins and minerals, which promote general health.
- **Food Groups:** To ensure a balanced nutritional intake, include all dietary groups—fruits, vegetables, proteins, carbohydrates, and dairy or dairy replacements.

2. Regular Eating Schedule:

- **Consistent Meals:** Maintain a consistent eating pattern of three meals and 2–3 snacks per day. This helps to maintain consistent energy levels and avoids excessive hunger.
- **Listen to Your Body:** Pay attention to your hunger and fullness cues, and aim to eat when you're hungry and stop when you're full.

3. Addressing Nutritional Gaps:

- **Supplementation:** Consider taking supplements as prescribed by a health-care practitioner to address particular nutrient shortages.

- **Professional Guidance:** Work with a trained dietitian to create a personalized eating plan that meets your specific nutritional requirements.

Enhancing Enjoyment

1. Trying new foods:

- **Variety:** Slowly incorporate new items into your diet. Begin with small servings and combine new meals with familiar, safe alternatives.
- **Flavor Experimentation:** Try new flavors, seasonings, and cooking ways to make meals more fun and appealing.

2. Mindful Eating:

- **Present Moment:** Focus on the current moment when eating. Pay attention to the flavor, texture, and scent of your food.
- **Savoring Each Bite:** Take your time with each bite, chewing carefully and enjoying the experience of eating.

3. Creating a Pleasant Dining Experience:

- **Atmosphere:** Make the dining area a relaxing and welcoming place. Set the table tastefully, play quiet music, or use lovely lighting to make eating more enjoyable.
- **Distraction-Free:** To completely focus on the eating process, keep distractions like television and phones to a minimum.

Combining nourishment with enjoyment.

1. Cooking and Preparing Meals:

- **Involvement:** Involve yourself in meal preparation and cooking. This can help you feel more connected to the food you consume and appreciate the experience more.
- **Fun Recipes:** Experiment with new recipes that fascinate you. Cooking may be a creative and pleasant hobby that enhances the pleasure of eating.

2. Social Eating:

- **Shared Meals:** Consider sharing meals with family or friends. Social connections during meals can make the dining experience more joyful and stress-free.
- **Positive Conversations:** During meals, engage in positive, uplifting conversations to foster a welcoming and supportive dining environment.

3. Food Celebrations:

- **Food Celebrations:** Recognise the importance of food in maintaining good health and wellness. View meals as an opportunity to nurture your body while also enjoying the sensory experience.
- **Cultural Traditions:** Discover and appreciate cultural eating customs. Trying meals from different cultures can provide diversity and delight in your diet.

Avoiding Food Rules and Restrictions

Food rules and limitations can worsen anxiety and limit the variety of foods consumed by people with ARFID (Avoidant/Restrictive Food Intake Disorder), resulting in additional nutritional deficits and a troubled connection with food. Avoiding these strict standards and instead taking a more flexible, intuitive approach to food can lead to a healthier, more balanced diet.

Understanding the impact of food regulations

1. Raised Anxiety and Fear:

- **Pressure and guilt:** Strict food regulations frequently produce pressure to eat correctly and feelings of shame when those rules are disobeyed, which heightens anxiety about eating.
- **Food Fear:** Labelling foods as "good" or "bad" can cause fear and avoidance of specific foods, restricting dietary variety.

2. Nutritional Imbalance:

- **Limited Food Choices:** Adhering to stringent eating guidelines can result in a monotonous diet devoid of key nutrients, and worsening nutritional deficits.
- **Missed Nutrients:** Avoiding entire food groups or types might result in a lack of essential vitamins, minerals, and other nutrients for overall wellness.

Embracing Flexible Eating

1. Allowing All Foods:

- **No Forbidden Foods:** Adopt the idea that no food is off-limits. This alleviates the fear and anxiety associated with eating and promotes a more diverse diet.
- **Incorporating Favourites:** Include favorite foods regularly in your diet, even if they are usually thought to be less healthful. This promotes a favorable relationship with eating.

2. Listen to Your Body:

- **Hunger and Fullness:** Recognize your body's natural hunger and fullness cues. Eat when you're hungry and stop when you're full, rather than following external guidelines.
- **Cravings and Preferences:** Honor your cravings and preferences. Eating what you appreciate can increase satisfaction and lessen the desire to overeat.

3. Mindful Eating:

- **Present Moment Focus:** Practice being completely present at meals, concentrating on the sensory experience of eating. This helps you become more aware of your body's demands and preferences.
- **Nonjudgmental Awareness:** Approach eating with a nonjudgmental mindset. Accept your eating choices without judging them as "good" or "bad."

Strategies to Avoid Food Rules

1. Challenge Restrictive Thoughts:

- **Question the rules:** When you discover restricted thoughts, challenge their veracity. Consider whether these restrictions are genuinely beneficial or if they increase tension and anxiety.
- **Reframe ideas:** Reframe negative food ideas by emphasizing the benefits of a diverse diet and the enjoyment of eating different foods.

2. Gradual Exposure to Fear Foods:

- **Small Steps:** Begin with little steps to gradually introduce fearful foods. Begin with modest amounts of fear foods and gradually increase as you get more comfortable. Reduce anxiety by pairing them with safe, familiar meals.

- **Positive Reinforcement:** Celebrate every step forward, no matter how tiny. Positive reinforcement promotes confidence and lessens fear over time.

3. Seeking Professional Support:

- **Therapeutic guidance:** Work with a therapist who specializes in eating disorders to treat the underlying anxiety and restrictive thought patterns caused by dietary rules.
- **Dietitian Assistance:** A qualified dietitian can assist you in developing a flexible eating plan that meets your nutritional requirements without imposing harsh rules or limits.

Developing a Positive Relationship with Food.

1. Food as nourishment and joy:

- **Balanced Perspective:** Think of food as more than simply fuel; it's also a source of nourishment and delight. Accept the sensory delights of eating and the advantages of a diverse diet.
- **Positive Experiences:** Try new recipes, dine with friends, or experiment with different cuisines to create enjoyable eating experiences.

2. Self-Compassion and Acceptance:

- **Be kind to yourself:** When it comes to eating, remember to be kind to yourself. Accept that having a variety of eating habits is acceptable and that perfection is not required.
- **Body Respect:** Honour your body's demands and cues. Trust that your body knows what it needs and can lead you to healthy, happy eating.

3. Celebrating Food Freedom:

- **Freedom from Rules:** Celebrate the freedom from restricted food rules. Enjoy the diversity and flexibility this provides for your diet.
- **Positive Mindset:** Develop a positive attitude towards food, emphasizing the benefits of a broad and balanced diet for your general health.

Preventing Relapse: Identifying Triggers and Developing Coping Mechanisms

Recognizing the stressors and triggers that increase symptoms is critical for treating ARFID (Avoidant/Restrictive Food Intake Disorder) and making progress in recovery. Stressors and triggers differ greatly among individuals, but understanding them is an important step in establishing successful coping techniques. Here's how to detect and comprehend these elements:

Common stressors and triggers

1. Sensory sensitivities:

- **Textures and scents:** Unfamiliar or unpleasant food textures and scents can cause aversions and anxiety, making certain foods difficult to consume.
- **Visual Appearance:** The appearance of food, including color and presentation, can be a powerful motivator.

2. Emotional Stress:

- **Anxiety and Depression:** Anxiety and despair can exacerbate ARFID symptoms, leading to avoidance of food and eating settings.
- **Stressful Life Events:** Major life events, such as relocation, school changes, or family concerns, can increase stress and have a detrimental impact on eating habits.

3. Social circumstances:

- **Eating in Public:** ARFID individuals may experience anxiety when eating in public or social settings, causing them to avoid such circumstances.
- **Social Pressure:** Pressure from family, friends, or peers to consume specific foods or eat more can exacerbate symptoms and contribute to stress.

4. Negative Experiences:

- **Previous Choking or Vomiting Incidents:** Previous choking or vomiting incidents might cause anxiety and avoidance of certain meals or eating in general.
- **Unfavorable Comments:** Criticism or unfavorable comments about eating habits or food choices can cause shame and anxiety, exacerbating ARFID symptoms.

5. Rigid Routines:

- **Strict Eating Schedules:** Strict eating patterns can cause stress when variations occur, making it difficult to adapt to new foods and settings.
- **Limited Food Preferences:** Relying on a small number of safe foods might cause anxiety when they are not accessible, leading to restrictive eating habits.

Strategies for identifying stressors and triggers

1. Self-Reflection and Awareness:

- **Food Diary:** Keep a food diary to record what you eat, how you feel before and after eating, and any circumstances that may have influenced your eating habits.

- **Emotional Check-Ins:** Regularly check in with yourself to detect any emotions or stressors influencing your eating patterns.

2. Identifying Patterns:

- **Common Themes:** Look for similar themes or trends in your food journal or emotional check-ins that could point to specific stressors or triggers.
- **Situational Analysis:** Examine specific situations where your ARFID symptoms worsen to uncover potential causes.

3. Professional Support:

- **Therapist Support:** Collaborate with a therapist who specializes in eating disorders to identify stresses and triggers.
- **Dietitian Input:** A certified dietician can help you understand how specific meals or eating patterns may be linked to stressors and triggers.

Managing identified stressors and triggers

1. Gradual Exposure:

- **Desensitization:** Desensitization involves gradually exposing oneself to triggering foods or events in a controlled and supportive atmosphere to minimize anxiety.
- **Modest Steps:** Begin with modest, controllable steps and progressively expand exposure as you gain comfort.

2. Stress Reduction Techniques:

- **Relaxation Practices:** To handle stress and anxiety, incorporate relaxation techniques like deep breathing, mindfulness, and meditation.
- **Healthy Coping Mechanisms:** Create healthy stress-management strate-

gies, such as physical activity, hobbies, or talking to a trusted friend or therapist.

3. Fostering a Supportive Environment:

- **Positive Support System:** Surround yourself with caring family, friends, or support groups who understand and respect your ARFID issues.
- **Open Communication:** Be honest with your support system about your triggers and stressors so that they may help create a more accommodating atmosphere.

4. Flexible Routines:

- **Adapting Routines:** Create flexible eating routines to decrease anxiety from strict timetables and limited meal selections.
- **Incremental modifications:** Make minor, incremental modifications to your eating habits to gradually broaden your variety of safe foods and minimize reliance on strict regimens.

5. Professional Treatment:

- **Therapy:** Treatment options include Cognitive Behavioural Therapy (CBT) and Exposure Therapy, which can effectively address anxiety and fear associated with ARFID.
- **Nutritional Counselling:** Meeting with a certified dietician regularly can provide continuous support and assistance for eating well while dealing with stress.

Developing Healthy Coping Mechanisms for Stress and Emotional Eating

For people with ARFID (Avoidant/Restrictive Food Intake Disorder), stress and emotional eating can have a big impact on their eating patterns and overall health. Developing healthy coping techniques is critical for overcoming these obstacles and cultivating a more balanced relationship with food.

Understanding Stress and Emotional Eating.

1. Stress Eating:

- **What It Is:** Stress Eating Stress eating is when you eat food because you're stressed or anxious, not hungry.
- **Impact:** This can lead to unhealthy eating habits, weight swings, and increased concern about food.

2. Emotional Eating:

- **What It Is:** Emotional eating is the use of food to alleviate negative feelings including melancholy, loneliness, and boredom.
- **Impact:** It can lead to feelings of guilt and shame, as well as a negative cycle of eating to cope with emotions.

Strategies to Develop Healthy Coping Mechanisms

1. Mindfulness and Self-awareness:

- **Identify triggers:** Keep a journal to track what causes your stress and emotional eating. Recognizing these tendencies will allow you to address them more effectively.

- **Mindful Eating:** Practice staying present during meals. Focusing on the taste, texture, and enjoyment of food might help minimize mindless eating.

2. Relaxation techniques:

- **Deep Breathing:** Deep breathing exercises might help relax your mind and body when you're anxious or emotionally overwhelmed.
- **Progressive Muscle Relaxation:** Tense each muscle group before progressively releasing it to relieve physical strain and stress.

3. Healthful Distractions:

- **Physical Activity:** Walking, yoga, or dancing can help you shift your focus and boost your mood, making exercise an effective stress reliever.
- **Creative Outlets:** To distract yourself from emotional eating, try hobbies or creative pursuits like painting, writing, or playing music.

4. Establishing a Support Network:

- **Contact Someone:** Communicate your feelings to a trustworthy friend, family member, or therapist. Talking about your emotions will help you feel better and minimize your need to eat for consolation.
- **Join Supporting Groups:** Connect with others who understand your struggles by joining ARFID support groups or online communities.

5. Setting Healthy Routines:

- **Regular Meals:** Establish a regimen of regular meals and snacks to avoid acute hunger, which can lead to stress eating.
- **Balanced Diet:** Make an effort to eat a diverse range of foods. This can assist ensure you get enough nutrients and prevent cravings.

6. Cognitive-Behavioral Techniques:

- **Challenge Negative Thoughts:** Identify and fight the negative ideas that contribute to emotional eating. Replace them with positive affirmations and realistic outlooks.
- **Behavioral Alternatives:** Make a list of non-food things to do when you have a want to eat due to stress or emotions. This could involve going for a walk, reading a book, or pursuing a hobby.

7. Self-Compassion and Acceptance:

- **Be kind to yourself:** Practice self-compassion. Recognize that everyone experiences emotional ups and downs, and it is acceptable to seek solace in non-food ways.
- **Accept imperfection:** Understand that it is appropriate to seek consolation from food on occasion. The goal is to create healthy behaviors over time, not to achieve perfection.

Implementing Coping Mechanisms

1. Start Small:

- **Gradual Changes:** Apply one or two strategies at a time. Gradual adjustments are more sustainable and manageable.
- **Celebrate Progress:** Recognise and celebrate minor successes. Each step forward represents development towards improved coping mechanisms.

2. Consistency is key:

- **Regular Practice:** Incorporate these coping strategies into your routine. The more consistently you practice, the more successful they will be.
- **Routine Adjustments:** Be adaptable and open to changing your strategies

as necessary. What works at one moment may need to be modified if your circumstances or stressors change.

3. Seek professional help:

- **Therapist Guidance:** A therapist can provide you with personalised methods and support as you seek to establish healthy coping skills.
- **Nutritional Counselling:** A licensed dietician can help you maintain a healthy diet and manage emotional eating triggers.

The Importance of Maintaining Treatment Gains Over Time

Making progress in treating ARFID (Avoidant/Restrictive Food Intake Disorder) is an important milestone, but maintaining those improvements over time is also critical. Sustained improvement promotes long-term health and well-being by preventing relapse and reinforcing healthy behaviors. Here's why it's important to preserve treatment gains and how to do so effectively:

Why Maintaining Treatment Gains is Important.

1. Long-term Health Benefits:

- **Nutritional Stability:** Eating a well-balanced diet consistently helps to prevent nutrient shortages, which benefits general physical health.
- **Growth and Development:** For children and adolescents, preserving treatment gains is critical to appropriate growth and development.

2. Emotional and Psychological Stability.

- **Reduced Anxiety:** Maintaining coping techniques minimizes anxiety and other negative emotions associated with eating.
- **Enhanced Self-Esteem:** Making steady progress gives you a sense of

success while also improving your self-esteem and body image.

3. Relapse Prevention:

- **Avoiding Setbacks:** Resuming old eating habits might reverse progress and trigger ARFID symptoms again.
- **Building Resilience:** Consistent practice of healthy behaviors strengthens resilience to stressors and triggers that can lead to relapses.

Strategies to Maintain Treatment Gains

1. Regular Monitoring and Check-ins:

- **Self-Monitoring:** Keep a journal to record your eating habits, emotions, and any obstacles you encounter. Regular self-reflection allows for the early detection of potential problems.
- **Professional Support:** Schedule regular follow-up meetings with your therapist, dietician, or doctor to track your progress and handle any new concerns.

2. Reinforcing Healthy Habits:

- **Consistent Routine:** Establish a regular eating routine with balanced meals and snacks. Routine helps to maintain stable eating habits.
- **Variety and Flexibility:** Continue to try different things and be adaptable to your diet. This prevents relapse into restrictive eating habits.

3. Ongoing Support:

- **Support Networks:** Stay in touch with support groups or internet communities. Sharing experiences and gaining positive feedback from others can be inspiring.

- **Family & Friends:** Maintain communication with your family and friends during your journey. Their support and understanding are critical for growth.

4. coping strategies for stress and triggers:

- **Stress Management:** Continue to practice stress-reduction practices including mindfulness, deep breathing, and physical activity.
- **Trigger Identification:** Be careful in recognizing and handling triggers. Develop and enhance ways of dealing with them effectively.

5. Set realistic short-term goals:

- **Short-Term Goals:** Set realistic short-term goals to keep you motivated and focused. Celebrate little triumphs to keep the enthusiasm going.
- **Long-Term Vision:** Consider your long-term health and well-being goals. Remind yourself regularly of the benefits of preserving treatment gains.

6. Flexible and Adaptable Strategies:

- **Adapting Strategies:** Be willing to alter your strategies as your circumstances change. Flexibility is essential for sustaining success over time.
- **Learning from Setbacks:** If you have setbacks, consider them learning opportunities. Analyze what caused the setback and how you can avoid it in the future.

7. Self-compassion and Positive Reinforcement:

- **Be kind to yourself:** Practice self-compassion. Recognize that maintaining development is a journey filled with ups and downs.
- **Positive Reinforcement:** Reward yourself for keeping healthy habits and achieving milestones. Positive reinforcement increases devotion to your goals.

Embracing Your Journey: Living a Fulfilling Life with ARFID

Living with ARFID (Avoidant/Restrictive Food Intake Disorder) can be difficult, but it's critical to identify and build on your skills and abilities. Focusing on your strengths and accomplishments can boost your confidence and promote a good attitude. Here's how to recognize, appreciate, and exploit your talents and capabilities during your ARFID journey:

Why Focusing on Strengths and Capabilities is Important.

1. Enhances self-esteem:

- **Positive Self-Image:** Recognising your strengths increases self-esteem and fosters a more positive self-image.
- **Confidence Building:** Recognising your strengths and successes boosts your confidence and motivation.

2. Promotes Resilience:

- **Coping Skills:** Drawing on your strengths allows you to establish effective coping techniques for dealing with ARFID-related issues.
- **Problem-Solving:** Focusing on capabilities improves your problem-solving talents, allowing you to traverse challenges more successfully.

3. Enhances Overall Well-being:

- **Emotional Health:** Recognising and utilizing your strengths improves emotional well-being while decreasing anxiety and stress.
- **Balanced Perspective:** Focusing on strengths gives you a balanced view, helping you to look beyond the constraints imposed by ARFID.

Strategies to Identify and Build on Strengths

1. Self-Reflection:

- **Personal Inventory:** Evaluate your skills, talents, and accomplishments. Make a list of your strengths, both food-related and not.
- **Acknowledge progress:** Consider the progress you've made in your ARFID journey. Recognize the minor successes and improvements you have made.

2. Feedback from Others:

- **Seek Input:** Seek feedback from trusted others, such as friends, family, or therapists, to gain insight into your skills. They may highlight features you haven't considered.
- **Positive Reinforcement:** Accept compliments and positive feedback gracefully. Use this reinforcement to boost your self-esteem.

3. Utilising Strengths in Daily Life:

- **Apply Skills:** Identify how you can use your abilities to tackle ARFID issues. For example, if you're skilled at organizing, utilize your skills to plan healthy meals.
- **Strength-Based Activities:** Participate in activities that allow you to use your strengths. This not only builds confidence but also gives a feeling of accomplishment.

4. Creating Realistic Goals:

- **Strength-Based Goals:** Set goals that are consistent with your strengths and capabilities. Achieving these targets strengthens your skills and develops momentum.

- **Incremental Progress:** Break down enormous ambitions into smaller, more doable steps. To stay motivated and confident, celebrate each accomplishment.

5. Building New Strengths:

- **Continuous Learning:** Develop new talents through continuous learning. This can involve cooking, relaxation techniques, and social skills.
- **Challenge Yourself:** Stepping outside of your comfort zone can help you build resilience and uncover new skills. Each additional skill adds to your strength arsenal.

6. Practice Self-Compassion:

- **Be kind to yourself:** Practice self-compassion and avoid self-criticism. Recognize that everyone has abilities and opportunities for development.
- **Embrace Imperfection:** Recognise that setbacks are normal. Focus on what you've learned and how you can use your strengths to move forward.

Practical tips for emphasizing strengths

1. Daily Affirmations:

- **Positive Affirmations:** Begin each day with affirmations that highlight your abilities. Like the following: "I am capable of making healthy food choices today."
- **Consistent Practice:** To stay positive, remind yourself of your strengths and accomplishments regularly.

2. Strength Journaling:

- **Strength Diary:** Keep a notebook to track your abilities, daily accomplishments, and pleasant experiences. Reviewing this notebook can help you stay positive throughout difficult times.

- **Reflective Writing:** Explain how you've used your strengths to overcome specific problems. This strengthens your abilities and gives a road map for future success.

3. Supportive Environment:

- **Encouragement:** Surround yourself with helpful others who acknowledge and celebrate your strengths.
- **Positive Feedback Loop:** Join communities or support groups where you may discuss your triumphs and get positive feedback.

Setting Goals Outside of Food and Eating

While dealing with ARFID (Avoidant/Restrictive Food Intake Disorder) typically necessitates focusing on eating habits and nutritional goals, it is also critical to establish goals that go beyond food and eating. These bigger goals can help you improve your general quality of life, give you a sense of purpose, and boost confidence. Here's how to discover and pursue non-food goals:

The importance of broader goals

1. Diversifying Focus:

- **Balanced Life:** Setting objectives outside of food can help you live a more balanced existence in which eating habits are just one aspect of your overall well-being.
- **Reduced burden:** It takes some of the burden off food-related progress, making the path less daunting.

2. Increased Self-Worth:

- **Building Confidence:** Achieving non-food-related goals strengthens your abilities and increases your self-esteem.
- **Positive Identity:** It allows you to perceive yourself as a whole person with diverse interests and strengths, rather than merely someone battling with an eating disorder.

3. Enhance Enjoyment and Fulfilment:

- **Pursuing Passions:** Pursuing enjoyable hobbies and goals can boost emotional well-being.
- **Personal Growth:** It offers possibilities for learning, growth, and personal development in areas that are important to you.

Identifying Non-Food-Related Goals

1. Reflect on Your Interests:

- **Hobbies and Passions:** Consider the hobbies you enjoy or have always wanted to do. This could be sports, arts, music, travel, or any other pastime.
- **Skill Development:** Consider what abilities you want to grow or improve, such as learning a new language, playing an instrument, or mastering a craft.

2. Focus on Relationships:

- **Social Connections:** Set goals for building and nurturing relationships with friends, family, and the community.
- **Volunteering:** Consider volunteering for issues that you care about. It can be rewarding and provide a sense of purpose.

3. Professional and academic goals:

- **Career Goals:** Determine what professional successes you wish to pursue, such as moving forward in your career, establishing a new job, or obtaining extra certifications.
- **Educational Goals:** Set educational goals, such as succeeding in your current academics, seeking higher education, or learning new disciplines.

Steps for Setting and Achieving Broader Goals

1. SMART goals:

- **Specific:** Clearly describe your goals. For example, "Learn to play three songs on the guitar."
- **Measurable:** Ensure that the aim is measurable. For example, "Read two books per month."
- **Achievable:** Set realistic, attainable goals. Begin small and gradually raise the challenge.
- **Relevant:** Select goals that are significant to you and reflect your values and interests.
- **Time-bound:** Determine a deadline for completing the goal. Like this one: "Join a community choir within the next three months."

2. Break Down Goals:

- **Step-by-Step Plan:** Create a step-by-step plan to break down goals into smaller, more doable ones. This makes the task less overwhelming and aids in progress.
- **Prioritise tasks:** Determine the most crucial steps and tackle them first.

3. Track your progress:

- **Regular check-ins:** Regularly assess your progress towards your goals. Adjust your plan as needed, and celebrate accomplishments along the way.

- **Accountability:** Share your goals with a trustworthy friend, family member, or therapist who can offer advice and motivation.

4. Be flexible:

- **Adapt and Adjust:** Be prepared to adapt your aims when the situation changes. Flexibility enables you to keep on track even when confronted with setbacks.
- **Learn from Setbacks:** If you have setbacks, view them as learning opportunities. Consider what went wrong and how you can overcome similar challenges in the future.

Examples of broader goals.

1. Physical activity:

- **Exercise routine:** Create a regular fitness program that you enjoy, like yoga, swimming, hiking, or dancing.
- **Fitness Goals:** Set particular fitness goals, such as completing a 5K, increasing strength, or learning a new sport.

2. Creative Activities:

- **Art Projects:** Express yourself via art projects such as painting, drawing, and making.
- **Writing:** Begin a journal, or blog, or concentrate on creative writing projects.

3. Personal Development:

- **Mindfulness Practices:** Practice mindfulness or meditation to alleviate stress and increase emotional well-being.

- **Time Management:** Improve your time management abilities to efficiently balance your life's numerous responsibilities.

4. Community Involvement:

- **Join groups:** Participate in clubs, organizations, or community groups that share your interests.
- **Local Initiatives:** Take part in local initiatives or events that are important to you.

Living a Rich and Fulfilling Life Despite ARFID

Living with Avoidant/Restrictive Food Intake Disorder (ARFID) presents considerable obstacles, but it does not have to define your life. With the correct tactics and mindset, you may live a rich and satisfying life despite ARFID. Here's how to take a comprehensive approach to well-being, emphasizing personal development, relationships, and appreciating life's numerous chances.

Adopting a Holistic Approach to Well-being

1. Prioritising Mental Health:

- **Therapeutic Support:** Seek regular treatment to treat anxiety, depression, and other emotional issues related to ARFID.
- **Mindfulness Practices:** Use mindfulness and relaxation practices to reduce stress and improve emotional equilibrium.
- **Self-Compassion:** Instead of criticizing yourself, practice self-compassion. Recognize that managing ARFID is a journey that includes setbacks.

2. Promoting Physical Health:

- **Regular exercise:** Discover physical activities that you enjoy. Exercise not only benefits your physical health, but it also boosts your mood and reduces anxiety.
- **Adequate Sleep:** Make sure you receive plenty of restful sleep every night. Good sleep hygiene is critical to overall health.
- **Balanced Nutrition:** Collaborate with a dietitian to develop a balanced meal plan that meets your nutritional requirements while respecting your dietary restrictions.

3. Fostering Social Connections:

- **Building Relationships:** Invest time in developing ties with family and friends. Strong social support can create motivation and a sense of community.
- **Joining Communities:** Engage in social groups, clubs, or online communities that share your interests. This can assist in alleviating feelings of loneliness and create a support system.

Pursuing Personal Development and Fulfilment

1. Set Meaningful Goals:

- **Personal Interests:** Identify hobbies and activities that bring joy and fulfillment. Set goals based on these interests, such as learning a new skill or pursuing a creative pastime.
- **Professional aspirations:** Concentrate on professional or academic objectives. Seek opportunities for advancement and development in your chosen field.
- **Volunteering:** Do volunteer labor or community service. Helping others can bring a sense of purpose and fulfillment.

2. Celebrating Achievements:

- **Acknowledging Progress:** Acknowledging Progress Regularly reflect on and celebrate your accomplishments, no matter how minor. Recognizing progress increases self-esteem and motivation.
- **Rewarding Yourself:** Give yourself rewards for achieving milestones. This can help you maintain positive behaviors and stay motivated.

3. Exploring New Experiences:

- **Travel and Adventure:** Explore new places and civilizations. Travel can broaden your perspective and bring rewarding experiences.
- **Trying New Activities:** Get out of your comfort zone by trying new activities or hobbies. This might lead to personal development and new interests.

Finding Joy and Meaning in Daily Life.

1. Practice Gratitude:

- **Daily Gratitude:** Keep a gratitude journal and write down what you're grateful for every day. This technique might help you focus on the positive parts of life.
- **Appreciating the Present:** Appreciate and relish the present moment. Mindfulness practices might help you stay grounded and enjoy ordinary activities.

2. Engaging in Creative Expression:

- **Art and Music:** Express yourself creatively through art, music, or writing. Creative expression may be both healing and satisfying.
- **Crafts and DIY Projects:** Try your hand at crafts or DIY projects. Making something with your hands may be both calming and satisfying.

3. Building Resilience:

- **Facing Challenges:** Consider challenges as chances for progress. Each hurdle overcome can boost your resilience and self-efficacy.
- **Learning from Setbacks:** Recognise that setbacks are a part of the process. Utilize them as learning opportunities to improve your strategies and approaches.

Conclusion

As we wrap up "Breaking Free from ARFID: A Compassionate Guide to Overcoming Eating Challenges," let's revisit the journey we've taken together. We've explored what ARFID is, its impact on daily life, and practical ways to manage and overcome it.

Understanding ARFID is crucial. It's more than just picky eating it's a serious condition that can affect anyone, at any age. Recognizing the symptoms and knowing how they differ from other eating issues is the first step toward dealing with them.

Seeking professional help is important. Early intervention from therapists, dietitians, and doctors can make a big difference. These professionals can help create a personalized plan to guide you through recovery.

Building a support network is key. Family and friends can provide the encouragement and understanding you need. Educating them about ARFID and involving them in your journey can make a significant impact.

We've discussed practical strategies to manage ARFID, such as exposure therapy, cognitive behavioral techniques, and mindfulness practices. These tools can help reduce anxiety, expand your food choices, and improve your relationship with food.

Self-compassion and acceptance are essential. Recovery is a journey with ups and downs. Celebrating small victories and setting realistic goals can keep you motivated and build resilience.

Remember, you are not alone. Connecting with others who understand your experience, through support groups or online communities, can provide additional strength and inspiration. Sharing your story and raising awareness can also be powerful steps in your healing process.

Breaking free from ARFID is possible. With the right knowledge, support, and determination, you can overcome its challenges and lead a fulfilling, healthy life. Take each step with hope and confidence, knowing that you are moving closer to a life where food is a source of nourishment and joy, not fear.

Thank you for allowing this book to be part of your journey. Here's to a brighter, healthier future one step at a time.